Warrior Princess

Undefeated

Warrior Princess Undefeated

My Life Living with Cancer

JACQUELINE RIDOUT

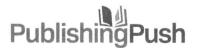
PublishingPush

First Edition 2022

ISBN 978-1-80227-280-2 (paperback)
ISBN 978-1-80227-281-9 (ebook)

Book cover photography by James Noble Photography

Illustrations by Jo Cooke-Best

Book design by Publishing Push

Published by PublishingPush.com

Typeset using Atomik ePublisher from Easypress Technologies

Prologue

Books of all kinds can take us through other's experiences, on an adventure or to a different place or time. We can relate to some stories and by reading them it helps us to understand and learn through someone else's eyes. Stories, whether fact or fiction, old or new, can be told and re-told differently over time to new generations.

It may have all been said before but, I want to share the knowledge I have learned, which saved my life, and the fact that research and medicine will continually evolve and improve for others in the future.

I have always been a storyteller with photographs and now I am telling my story with words to share my individual experience. I want this book to be a therapeutic and enlightening read for people and to give the reader an insight from a very personal perspective of what happened to me; because behind every person there is a story to tell and this is my story, my personal journey and this is the most crucial point in my life.

Cancer, once diagnosed, never leaves you. Cancer brings clouds into a person's blue skies. Luckily for me, my cloud had a silver lining, and I was determined to get the sunshine back.

Since the beginning of my ordeal, I have kept a journal of my experience to give me an outlet, and to help me focus throughout. In writing this journal, it helped me to understand more about people who live with cancer and the hurdles they and their loved ones' face. I began to record everything that was going on in my journal and as time went on and my journal became bigger, I decided to keep going with it and write it as a book to share my story.

I feel that such information is not always something that is very forthcoming from cancer patients or doctors, and this is possibly because people with cancer are not always willing to share very personal experiences with the world.

As I will keep stressing throughout this book, we are not all the same and every individual's experience will be quite different. Therefore, what a doctor can see going on with one patient will not be the same for the next. They can only advise on what to expect during treatment, or what "could" happen.

I have written this book in the hope it will help others going through cancer, or those watching someone going through cancer or similar circumstances. My story, although harrowing for me, is one from a positive perspective and how I chose to live and not let go of hope.

Cancer is something I will live with for the rest of my life. It started in 2016 and lasted over a three-year period, from the point of diagnosis to making it to my fiftieth birthday – something at the time of being diagnosed that I never thought possible.

Along the way there have been some fascinating people who have loved me, comforted me, inspired me, and helped me to fight this all the way. These people who have been on this ride with me do not realise how brave they have been through all this and how special each of them are to me.

My immediate family, my parents and brother, are my world. They mean everything to me, and I love them more than life itself. They keep my spirits high and my heart beating stronger than ever. Amongst all this heartache and the tears, they have also kept the laughter on tap, which has been a good shock absorber to the blows in our lives.

I don't have a husband or kids, so I guess for me, this was one stress I didn't have to cope with.

I could not have done this without the support of my entire family (and a large one at that). It hit them much harder than I ever imagined but they all stood by me throughout. We are a close family and having to tell them once I was diagnosed, was one of the toughest things I had to do; much tougher than hearing that I had cancer.

My friends and work colleagues are my rocks and it amazed me the amount of people who reached out to me and were there for me at a time when I needed them most. I am truly fortunate in life to have the most amazing people in it.

The hospital staff in Southampton, without whom I would probably not be sitting here writing this book now - I do not know how they do their job helping people like me day in, day out. I see how dedicated they are to their patients and their jobs, and these people have done outstanding things in their encouragement, my treatment plan, and my ongoing care.

Then there are those in the public eye who I have admired from afar. People whose work I love such as musicians, actors, photographers, TV and sports personalities. Some tell their stories on TV or via a magazine article to highlight their cancer experiences and there are those who are more private, but who you may hear of in the media. I am also inspired by those who may not have experienced or shared their personal journeys in the media but whose movies and music carried me through a very dark time.

You see, there are many people from all walks of life that have given me understanding, strength, knowledge, and encouragement to keep going, keep smiling and keep living.

Hearing someone else's story can play such a big part in helping you to understand and overcome things like an illness and make you see that you are never alone.

I feel very blessed to have such amazing people in my life and I thank you all for giving me the strength to fight, the willpower to live and the empowerment to use what I can to spread the word and support and share the love to others. I want to give others hope and the determination to want to keep going, as you have all done for me.

With love from your Wonder Woman, your Warrior Princess, and sometimes your little pain in the rear end!

xx

* * *

Chapter One

Family

"It's cancer".

No one ever expects to hear this kind of news in their lifetime however, I did, and this is my story.

My name is Jacqueline. I was born and still live in Southampton in Hampshire, and I am living with cancer.

Cancer is something I feel people should never feel scared to talk about. It is a subject some people tend to shy away from. I do not, and I welcome anyone who broaches the subject with me.

Hopefully, this book will inspire someone else going through this and will help them to live with cancer and get through it as positively as possible.

I am an optimist and drawing on the support of my loved ones to get me through this has helped me a great deal.

Twice since 2016 I had cancer and I was given chemotherapy at hospital to combat it. Unfortunately for me, it is not curable but with ongoing maintenance treatment the medical team can help control it.

My first encounter with cancer in my body was back in January of 2002 when I was diagnosed with cancerous cells in my cervix and admitted to hospital for laser surgery to have the cells burned away.

This is now a much more commonly known thing for women to have done and is more widely spoken about. Since this small operation,

I have been a very fit and healthy person and my cervical smear results have all been clear.

The good side of having a cervical screening is that if done regularly and not avoided then if cancer is present, it can be caught at an early stage and dealt with. It is so important for our health to ensure we get these regular checks done.

With ovarian cancer, it is very unfortunate that it is not so easy to detect there is not a specific test for it. It is not something that can be picked up in routine screening like a cervical smear test and therefore it can grow without us ever knowing. Ovarian cancer can grow at an aggressive rate before it is detected or becomes noticeable within the body that there is something wrong. I was not going to take this news lying down and I intended to be around for a long time to come. Well, I had this book to finish for starters and then there is my 50th birthday to celebrate and I am certainly not one to miss out on a good party!

My glass is always half full and as the saying goes, I hope with the many life experiences I have had, that I will go to my grave skidding in sideways with a margarita in hand, a little ruffled round the edges, but with no regrets. I am enjoying life and I am not ready to give up the ghost just yet.

I have never been a wealthy person, yet I consider myself rich in life with the most amazing friends and family who I love unconditionally. We are a large family and over the years we have made many memorable moments together: holidays, party celebrations and family gatherings. We live life to the full and make the most of what we have.

My family have played such an important part in my journey with cancer, so I am going to tell you a little about them.

My dad grew up in Poppy Road, one of the flower roads in Southampton. He was one of five children to Ethel and Walter Ridout and baby brother to his four older sisters, Brenda, Edna, Margaret, and Doris. Dad was always the quieter of the clan and more laid back and being the only boy to four sisters they probably did most of the talking.

Mum's upbringing was quite different to my dad's. My grandmother left her husband, Grandad Loader, and their two young children. My grandad needed to continue to work to make a living and had no choice but to have them cared for so he could do this, and so my mum and Uncle Brian were sent on separate paths. Brian went to live with my grandad's relatives in Dorset, whilst mum, unbeknown to her dad, became a modern-day Cinderella for her aunt and uncle, working all the hours God sends.

Mum lived out this life until a time when she was of school leaving age, when she could afford to leave home and spread her wings in the big wide world. This was the time when she got herself a little flat and began to really start living.

My parents met whilst working for GM Motors, a world-wide company, at a Southampton based factory called AC Delco. Dad started working in the factory in 1956, and thereafter my mum got a job also working on the production lines. They became friends and it was not many years before their friendship blossomed into something more. I think the many pranks my mum played on my dad heavily contributed.

One day my mum trotted off to make a tea round with her friend and whilst walking back through the factory she noticed my dad bent over a machine trying to fix it. Mum could see his jeans stretched away from his backside and as she walked past him, she took the hot tea bags from the cups and threw them down the back of his trousers. They still laugh about it now and the fact that my mum had never seen my dad move so fast off his chair.

Another time dad left his workstation and whilst he was gone my mum got up to her usual mischievous tricks; she walked over to his chair and stuffed sheets of newspapers underneath. She waited for his return, and once he had sat back down, she crept up behind him and set light to the newspaper. It took a few minutes for my dad to feel the warmth to his backside to the extent he realised it was too hot to handle and he again jumped up off his chair swearing and cussing whilst behind he was being laughed at by mum and their work colleagues. They have both retained a good sense of humour and this has certainly helped me over the last three years.

Once my younger brother, Tony, and I came along, my mum gave up her job to look after us and my dad took a new role at the plant as a security officer. Although my brother and I are the spark in our parent's lives, through time there have been various incidents which occurred that probably gave my parents many a grey hair and wrinkle. Life was never dull in our family.

It didn't help on the stressful day of their house move from their start up home in an area called Sholing to their new "forever home", a twenty-minute ride away. That day they forgot something particularly important … Tony. He was seven years old at the time. My parents hadn't told him he needed to wait at school so they could pick him up. He came out, realised they were not there and so he walked back to our old house. At the front door he stood, and knocked hard to be let in, to then be greeted by some unfamiliar faces. The new occupiers were quick to contact my parents and told them of the horror on his poor little face at seeing them. A typical Home Alone movie scenario. Another time he was playing, and a desk fell on his leg. It became serious and for weeks after he had to have his leg injected regularly to prevent infection spreading.

Me? … Well, I wasn't only the attention seeker of the family, but also the accident prone one. Wherever there was trouble you can guarantee I was involved somehow. Like the time I held my breath when I couldn't get my own way until I keeled over on a pavement in the city centre, hit my head hard on the concrete, and had to be rushed to hospital. And then later when I was nine years old, my neighbour, Paula, and I decided to ride our bikes out of our cul-de-sac and three miles to another estate. Our bike ride took us to a park where a family football match was taking place on the adjacent field. I fell into a sandpit face down hitting my head hard. As I stood up reality hit as I noticed blood dripping from my head and then I saw what looked like pieces of a broken glass in the sandpit. There was a large protruding shard of green coloured glass sticking out of the sand covered in blood – my blood. I had cut my eyelid open. A few centimetres the wrong way and I would have lost my eye for sure.

In a panic Paula grabbed one of the dads watching the football match and before I knew it, he whisked me up in his arms and drove me straight to my parents, who then raced me to the hospital to be stitched up.

One time my dad had to swing by his local social club. Whilst dad was inside the club, Tony and I went over to play on the swings. To this day I am not sure why I did it, but I placed some coins I had into my mouth and as I swung back on the swing, I accidentally swallowed a 5 pence coin. These coins were just over 2cm in diameter back then. Yep, you guessed it ... another trip to A&E. The coin showed up clear as day on the X-ray, and the doctor reassured us that nature would take its course and it would leave my body naturally. I never saw that bloody coin again.

We certainly made life interesting for our parents.

Generally, life has been good to us, but it has not always been a bed of roses and for some in our family, life has been very tough. You cannot have the highs without the lows unfortunately and that is all part of life's little journey. It can be hard enough at the best of times for a lot of people, but it is about how we each choose to deal with our own circumstances and what life throws at us.

Whilst I am still alive and kicking, I choose to live life to the full no matter how long I might have left. Yes, I admit I am scared about having cancer, and I understand it can show itself to me again at any time. No, I do not wish to die; however it is inevitable that we all leave this planet eventually - I just do not believe my time is right now.

I do not go to church, unless attending celebrations such as weddings or christenings but, there are many times that I pray to God to be well and healthy. I pray that this will not affect my family too much and we can all be strong for each other and battle our way through this.

Past illnesses which affected my loved ones resonate a great deal with me. Both sides of my parent's family have experienced cancer, leukaemia and other life-threatening incidents and we have lost many loved ones along the way. The heartache we carry and the loss in our lives have only made us all much stronger and more resilient. Even with all the ailments my older aunties and uncles suffered, they each continued to live, laugh, and love their way through life. They totally inspired me for different reasons. They would go through the trauma, pain, and loss, yet would get on with it, making more memories with those around them.

I remember in the seventies when I was young; the family getting together often and having the most awesome times. We would all be celebrating on Boxing Day every year at a different family household. Back then there would be about 30 of us, give or take. The children would be put upstairs to bed as the evening grew late, whilst the adults continued partying into the early hours. Eventually the women would go to bed topping and tailing, and the men would retire to the living room with their playing cards, whisky bottle and sleeping bags and they would generally stay up until around 5:00 in the morning.

My brother and I were sometimes woken with the sound of laughter coming from the bedrooms and normally because my mum would be playing practical jokes on my aunties whilst they were each getting ready for bedtime, or she would stuff things under the covers to frighten my aunties when they got into bed. Complete nutters the lot of them, but these were some of the funniest memories.

The whole family would holiday together each year taking a ferry crossing from Southampton over to the Isle of Wight. We would stay at a holiday camp called Nodes Point.

This holiday consisted of dad's parents, mum's dad and all the aunties, uncles, and cousins. I remember our terraced chalet accommodation, and we all resided in chalets either next door to each other or a few chalets apart. I remember evenings in the onsite club house where they would hold various themed events for both adults and children. One night my mum, who has never smoked, won the sexiest smoker competition. She took a cigarette, casually walked up to the judges table, and as she perched her bottom on the end of the table, she put the cigarette into her mouth and lit it. Mum was always up for a good laugh, and she is the one I get my humour from.

Once, my dad and my uncles were roped into performing a balloon dance. To do this they stuffed blown up balloons under their shirts and had ties wrapped around their heads as they all broke out into a dance together.

Total nutters my family but I would not have them any other way.

Every year the campsite held a crepe paper fancy dress competition for the kids and each year our costumes would get better and better. One year the aunties helped to dress one of my cousins as a mermaid. It was not until after they completed her tail, wrapping various coloured crepe paper around her legs and adding the finishing touches to the costume, when they sat back and broke out in fits of laughter. They realised at that moment that my cousin couldn't walk, and mum still recalls how they tried to pick her up and carry her across the campsite, without splitting the crepe paper wrapped around her body. Memories like this are priceless.

There was an on-site shop that sold large pieces of honeycomb in packets. Every time I was given pocket money to spend, I would head there to purchase some. I can still remember how the texture felt as I broke a brittle piece off and placed it on my tongue to feel it bubble and melt into a sweet tasting sticky goo. I have so many memories of riding horseback up and down the embankment by the chalets, Grandad Ridout making kites out of newspapers and successfully flying them, my uncle John going cockling at the beach and then coming back sitting outside the chalet to soak them in large buckets. He would spend so much time prepping them. He would boil them and then put then into large jars to pickle them; they always tasted much better than the shop bought ones. Now every time I see jars of cockles on the supermarket shelves, they remind me of our Isle of Wight holidays.

In the mornings my grandad would be sat at the table and over on the tableside would be a glass of water with his false teeth soaking. This amusingly magnified them to look a lot larger than their true size. I remember one day particular day mum was dishing up the breakfast, and she turned around holding the frying pan to look at him. Then, with a straight face she asked grandad if he wanted his eggs on his plate or put in the glass with his false teeth.

There were times over there when all the family would get glammed up for the evening to go across to the club house, or we would get ready and traipse down to the local beach with cool bags and blankets in tow. Mum always made an excuse to stay behind a bit. Suddenly she would appear, or reach into her bag for something, and turn around in serious conversation wearing a funny Groucho Marx style face mask, or she would turn up wearing items of clothing she had pinched from various family members' chalets. The laughter erupted and as always, my aunties would start running to find the nearest toilets for fear of wetting themselves from laughing too much.

So, you see, my story is about the lowest point in my life, yet it feels right to share a fraction of the highs.

The poignant bit about writing this for me is to show my battle in a positive light, and to hopefully help people to understand that there is hope and that no matter what life throws at you, no matter how bad, heart-breaking, or stressful it might feel to you, I think you must try and give it your best shot.

At the time of being told I had ovarian cancer, I didn't know what timespan my life had left, yet over 3 years later I am still here today, living my life and appreciating every moment I have on this earth. It can be tough for a person going through an illness, yet it can be even tougher after an illness and having severe treatment inflicted on your body.

We are all uniquely different and not one experience will be the same to the next. Every person will have different feelings, deal with situations differently, have a different thought process and outlook on it all. Things like this can scare the hell out of most people because it is the unknown of what will be. And people going through such trauma will either crumble and feel like giving up or they will deal with it head on.

I want this book to show people that although I was feeling scared, I did not give up. It was hard for me at first and still is at times, but I am living proof that I conquered that fear. For me, cancer will always be there in both my body and mind. It cannot be removed, but I will continue to take medications to keep it supressed and prevent it spreading.

When I found out I had cancer, I was happy to speak openly about it with people, yet those who had experienced something like a hysterectomy operation, or the same type of cancer as me, whether it be themselves or a family member, would say, "Oh yeah, I had a hysterectomy and this is what it will feel like …" and would then talk to me about it as if they knew exactly what my pain was going to be. They did not! My pain was my pain. They didn't know how or what I was feeling.

Having a hysterectomy is not a nice operation to have done, I get that. I think it is totally different for someone like me, who has been cut from the belly button right down to the pelvic bone area, had their stomach opened and had cancerous tumours the size of tennis balls, plus all the masses, removed from parts of the stomach, and then a full hysterectomy, along with chemotherapy to try to rid my body of the disease. They literally took everything away: my ovaries, fallopian tubes, cervix, womb, etc. A hysterectomy alone for any woman is a hard-enough thing to accept, and yet I didn't care about that. I was having this operation done to save my life and to be honest, having a hysterectomy was the best thing I could have done.

Yes, people can relate to what you are going through, yes, they can empathise with you, and it is good to talk, share our experiences with each other and learn from each other. Many people will want to tell you, "Oh, I've had that done, you will be fine," or "you will feel like this". People probably say these things to be supportive and try to help the person going through cancer feel better about it. In some cases, it is not always what the person going through an illness wants to hear or will even experience themselves.

Often people on the outside looking in can feel very helpless or worry about what to say, or what not to say. There's no right or wrong way in all this, it can just feel difficult and sometimes stressful for those watching it happen, especially if the person going through the illness does not talk much about it. Anyone going through an illness will have a completely different experience and outlook to the next. A different level of pain threshold, tiredness, sickness, recovery time, body changes, etc.

People who go through any illness or trauma in their life will have their own individual experience. You can listen to others about what they have been through as this can give you an insight as to what the journey you are about to embark on could be like but, it will not be the same.

I heard stories and stumbled upon websites at times which scared me, but I was always mindful whilst gaining knowledge, to also not take everything as gospel. Our individual experiences and pain are each different and not just whilst going through it all. We are each affected post illness and post ops very differently too, and sometimes this can also change a person mentally as well as physically.

There will be people who do not fully understand the aftermath of how you feel on the inside and how your body is working twenty-four/seven to stay alive. They can only imagine what that person could be feeling or experiencing. Aesthetically, to look at me, you would never know there was anything wrong. I look like an extremely healthy person. People do not see what goes on behind the scenes; they only see what is on the outside.

Trust me, I now notice I am constantly dehydrated and, after a couple of alcoholic drinks on a night out with friends I can feel my organs working harder than ever to recoup. My heart starts to race, my temperature yoyos up and down, I feel slight pain to the kidney area. I do not even have to go to the pub and have a skinful these days to feel how my body is affected. Some people don't realise how quickly I now start to feel tired or sick from my drugs and will say "just have one more drink" or "just stay out a bit longer". I have learned when you are the person going through it, that it is entirely your call and if you become tired or feel unusual in yourself, then you need to SPEAK OUT and those around you who care enough should LISTEN and understand and allow you to do what you know is best for you.

I have only experienced a couple of incidents where people didn't listen to me and still wanted to come and visit me when I felt awful and I needed rest, or stay out to have that one more glass of wine before they were ready to take me home, even though they said they would ensure they would leave when I needed to go home, or they would change arrangements to suit them rather than me.

These were just minute niggles that happened, but mainly because these people still saw me as being outwardly the same. Happy Jackie, being strong, independent, enjoying life, and as I continued to get better, I looked so healthy to people, even though inside I felt, and can still feel, the struggle at times.

Before all this started with my illness, I feel I was a bit of a yes girl. Too often generous with money, happy to drive places, dropping plans to instantly be there for people who needed me. I know I am at fault for allowing myself to be treated this way and so certain people just expected it of me.

Having this illness has been a big wake up call for me and it has made me look at my life and relationships with people a lot differently. I consider myself more now when making decisions, and I spend my time, money, and energy making plans with those who do care, want to spend time with me, and put themselves out for me occasionally

Before all this I was literally burning myself out and had left myself with very little "me time". Maybe this was a contributor to the state of my health deteriorating. I think more now about my wellbeing, and I have become more of a no girl. I am less tolerant to those who constantly moan about trivial things. I will not put myself out like I used to, and I will sometimes sit back and wait for others to make the plans. Although I love to socialise a lot and love a good party, I realise more now that I am key, and my happiness and my health are so much more important to me. I spend more time in my own company with rest and self-love and appreciate what I have in life.

Chapter Two

Gut Instinct

It all started after my forty seventh birthday in mid May 2016. I had just started my new job. My stomach was becoming quite bloated to the extent I realised something wasn't right. I had a feeling as though I was getting constipated. I said to myself, there's no point going to the doctors, when I can sort this out myself with over-the-counter medication. I am not one to go to my GP for ailments that seem as trivial as a cold, when there are plenty of shop bought drugs and aids to help with such things. I decided to treat this myself so, for around two weeks I did what I thought was the right thing by taking laxatives and suppositories.

Well, I mean, it was constipation I was experiencing, right? … Just how wrong could I have been.

By end of May my stomach looked a lot larger, and I experienced the constant feeling of wanting to pee. When I lay on my side in bed it felt unusually sore and uncomfortable. This was beginning to frustrate me. It could probably be a wee infection, or bad constipation that was resting on my bladder and giving me the urge of needing to pee. Whatever it was, I didn't like it and I wanted this aggravation sorted.

The week commencing May 30th I walked into my GP surgery on the off chance of getting a walk-in appointment to see a doctor, or at least a nurse, to do some tests on me. The receptionist confirmed there was a nurse available, and I was able to be seen within 15 minutes of arriving at the surgery.

The nurse asked me a few general questions about how long I had been feeling like this? And what difficulties I was having, etc.? She asked me to wee in a sample bottle so she could run a dip stick test on my urine. Once she had finished testing me, the nurse said this all looked fine to her.

"This does seem to me like you do have constipation, so I suggest you go home and eat lots of high fibre in your diet. If you still feel like this in a couple of weeks, then you will need to make another appointment to see a doctor."

I sat in thought for a bit feeling confused and a little frustrated. I guess I expected to be advised differently rather than told to go home and eat a diet full of high fibre foods.

"I understand what you're saying to me, and although I think it could be constipation too, this feels somewhat different. It feels like there's something inside me; I can't explain it, but I can feel it when I try to lay on my side at night, like I'm lying on a hard tennis ball or something."

That was my gut instinct and the only way I could describe this feeling to the nurse.

The nurse looked at me and said, "I'm sure this is constipation. We have no available appointments, but do you want me to nip out to see if there's a doctor that may be free to talk with you in between appointments? ... it will be brief".

"Yes, if you could please; it would put my mind at rest, because what I'm feeling at the moment is different from when I have been constipated in the past, plus it feels quite sore and achy."

At this response, the nurse walked out of the medical room to see if there was a doctor available to talk with me. I sat there in her office for a few minutes, waiting patiently, with hope that a doctor would become available to chat to me, as I really didn't want to have to put up with this uncomfortable pain for much longer. A few minutes passed and then the nurse returned to the room. Unfortunately for me, there was no doctor available at that time, so I thanked the nurse for her time and left the surgery and did as she advised.

Straightaway I introduced more high fibre foods. Another two weeks passed, and I was becoming more and more uncomfortable. My stomach had grown a lot bigger in size and my natural concave body shape was now becoming more convex looking. I was eating less as I was worried about being unable to go to toilet, and I might do my body more harm than good if I kept stuffing it with food. As I lay there in bed at night, if I turned to sleep on my side I could feel an uncomfortableness to my stomach like it was stretched and taut. The sore feeling to my lower stomach as I rolled over in bed was still there, pressing inside, just above my groin area. It still felt as though I was laying on something hard, and I felt the need to want to push it away but couldn't.

This all came to a head when I took a drive out to visit my parents at their home. I parked my car on their driveway, took my handbag from the passenger seat and made my way through the garden gate to the back door. I tapped on the door, opened it, and made my way through the kitchen to the living room. As I entered the living room, the shock on mum and dad's faces when they saw the size of me just said it all. They looked horrified because I looked as though I was ready to give birth. I guess being a size eight and then looking like I was about to drop a full-term baby was a huge shock to them.

"Jac you really need to get back to the doctors and get this sorted, this isn't right. You look pregnant; we can see you aren't yourself, something's wrong," mum said.

Dad agreed and they were also puzzled as to why the nurse would send me away thinking it was constipation. Because this had suddenly happened over a couple of weeks, I guess the nurse came to the obvious conclusion, as did I. It wasn't as if I'd been showing a slow growth change in my body shape for months. BANG ... it just happened.

I looked at my parents and could see their concern.

"I know mum, and I've done as the nurse at my GP advised by eating a high fibre diet. It doesn't seem to be helping the issue and in fact I can see it's been getting worse. I'm too scared to eat too much food now, as I'm worried that I could have a reflux or an infection of some kind if it all starts backing up in my system."

Again, they stressed and pushed me to ensure I go back to my GP and get more tests done.

Dad said, "you can't leave this any longer Jac. Make sure you get an appointment as soon as you can and let us know how you get on".

I stayed at their place for quite a while, spending time chatting, until I decided it was time to be heading home.

After my visit to my parents, I realised this wasn't great and there was something seriously wrong that needed the urgent attention of my GP.

Lying in bed that night I was still thinking about how my parents had reacted to the sight of me. As I turned over to lay on my side, I had that feeling again as if I were laying on something, like a ball or stone. I knew I had to get this looked at immediately.

That very next morning I awoke and decided to go with what was my initial gut instinct two weeks previously, and I got in touch with my local surgery and made an appointment. I was booked to attend surgery to see Dr Roach on June 10th, 2016.

"Do you have anything sooner please?"

"No we don't but you can take this appointment and try calling before this date to see if we should have a cancellation."

I went ahead and took the appointment. Unfortunately, for me, nothing came up in the meantime.

In hindsight, I should have walked into my GP and demanded to be seen or got a second opinion elsewhere. I have heard that same story from many people that don't do this. They don't want to seem pushy or go with their gut instinct in case it's something trivial. They don't want to feel like they're wasting their GP's time in case it is nothing to warrant an appointment.

Knowing what I know now, I say just do it! Go with your initial feelings, trust that gut instinct and get yourself checked out. Don't leave it until it is too late. I would go straight away every time now, without fail, even if I'm not one-hundred percent sure. I don't care now if I feel like it could be a waste of time. That is what the GP surgery is there for. Be persistent if you must and get that appointment made.

There are many things I cannot stress enough to people, and this is one of them. People need to realise the importance and if you are not happy with what you are first told and still feel there is something wrong, then get a second opinion. This is not about being unable to trust what you have first been told, but about ensuring you deal with what is playing on your mind until you are satisfied, and if this means a second opinion elsewhere to do so, then this is better than leaving it and living with the stress and worry which only make things worse.

Thursday, June 16th at 17:10: thank goodness the time had come to get to my doctors for my diagnosis of what really was wrong with me, and hopefully get this uncomfortable feeling sorted out.

I got to the surgery and waited for no more than ten minutes.

"Jacqueline Ridout." "Yes.", I got up from the chair in the waiting area and was greeted by Doctor Roach.

"Hello Jacqueline, come on through."

I followed Dr Roach to her office. She turned and smiled, "how are you?"

I smiled back and replied, "yeah, fine", but that wasn't what I was actually feeling. We reached her room and she asked me to take a seat as she closed the door behind me. We started talking about my symptoms and then I got asked a series of questions. Doctor Roach wanted to check my stomach.

"Jacqueline come over here and lay face up on the bed for me, I need to feel around your tummy."

Dr Roach pulled up my top to view my stomach area and asked me to pull my waistband to my skirt down slightly so she could examine me. I watched the concentration in her face as she pressed and felt around my tummy and pelvic area.

No sooner had the doctor begun feeling around than she commented that she did not like what she could feel. It literally took her seconds to determine what she thought it could be. Dr Roach continued to feel around a bit more, and then she adjusted my clothing and asked me to sit up and to make my way back to sit on the chair by her desk. I did so, wondering what she was about to tell me.

My GP said, "I'm going to organise for you to have blood tests done back here at the surgery, and I will get an ultrasound scan booked in on the system now for you to attend the hospital. These appointments can have a long lead time so I will fast track this through for you".

She advised me that this did feel like a growth in my stomach area, and she needed me to have my bloods done and then attend the hospital for further tests for exact confirmation as to what kind of growth it was and if the growth might be benign or malignant.

"How big are they because I can feel them when I lay on my side?"

Dr Roach looked at me and said, "I'm not sure exactly, but you do have what feels like large cysts. The sooner we get your appointments started then the sooner we can determine what the next step will be, Jacqueline".

I sat in shock. I wasn't expecting to hear this, and I became a little worried as to what this could now lead to (or not, as I was hoping the case would be). My doctor, although showing great concern about this, was very reassuring and she acted immediately in getting the ball rolling with my appointments to see a specialist.

Once I left my doctors surgery, I contacted my parents to let them know the score. Next on my list was to call my boss, Jo, and let her know. At this stage it was still uncertain as to what it was but at the same time, it still felt unsettling as it was the unknown. Both Jo and I agreed that until we knew what it was, there was no point in worrying too much.

Jo has been so supportive in all this, and although she had to see things from a business point of view, she also took on board how I must have been feeling and what a stressful time this was for me going for tests and waiting to hear back. I discussed every appointment I had with her and regularly kept her up to date as to what had been said and when the next hospital visits were to take place, and Jo managed all the reception cover in my absence from work so that I didn't have the worry of this. For me, knowing that work was covered was such a huge weight lifted from me and I could focus on the bigger picture.

The next day at work I carried on about my day. My colleague asked how my appointment went and I explained the conversation I had with my GP.

She said "Jackie, it probably isn't what you think it is and they're just following procedure".

This, I was very much hoping, was the case. Once settled, I walked up the stairs to make a drink. I popped my head in on the girls upstairs and we had a chat about it. My colleagues have always been understanding, supportive and lifted me at times when I needed it. The team had not known me long, yet I felt the togetherness and comradery between us all. They are good people that care, and it takes the stress off, knowing my colleagues also have my back.

Jo arrived at work and asked to speak with me in the meeting room. I explained everything again to her so that she could update the management team.

"Now Jackie, it is early stages and although we hope it is not what you feel it might be, try to stay focused at work and positive until you can find out more. The less stressed you are in your body and mind, the better. We need to keep you well and looked after."

Jo was saying all the right things, she reined me in when things got tough, and she kept me on track thinking positively. She has a bit of a' tough cookie' side to her, probably because she has the responsibility of keeping the workplace running on all cylinders, but that woman certainly has a heart of gold to go with it.

The following Monday I had my CA125 blood tests done back at my local GP surgery. These tests were to check the levels of protein in my red blood cells. A normal result would be under thirty-five, anything rising over this sends alarms bells ringing.

A high rise in blood proteins can mean several things ranging from serious illnesses to being some other kind of activity like a cold, menstruating, endometriosis or irritable bowel issue. The protein rise in the blood doesn't always mean cancer; it means activity is going on within your body, which makes it harder to say for certain if it is cancer without having a follow up scan to determine all this. Due to there being tumour growths in my body (that seemed a dead cert now), the doctor needed to be sure if these were cancerous, and it would be the levels of protein that would determine this and the path we would be taking with going for further tests.

During this week, I noticed I was starting to feel a shortness of breath and pains to the left side of my chest. My stomach felt very sore to touch or when I moved. There was a constant pressing feeling to my bladder, and less bowel activity. I found as time went on and things got worse, I was writing lists ready to take to doctor or hospital appointments to show them what was happening and when. These lists had such things noted as bad pains and indigestion that felt like trapped wind, bloating, hard stomach, waking regularly throughout the night to wee, straining to go to toilet, and slight bleeding when I did manage to go. I experienced a rise in my temperature which made me feel extremely hot quickly and more often, and I suffered more with my eczema, although not sure that is anything to do with my cancer, but more of a stress factor causing my skin inflammation. I just wanted to ensure that I told my doctors everything in case any of this could indicate what was happening to my body and help them understand. I put questions to paper as they came to mind, such as: should I stop taking the pill? Could I use certain laxatives regularly like Senokot, Fibre Gel or suppositories?

I began to also start drinking nutrient shakes for my lunch so that I didn't go hungry. I felt this would be better for me to drink something rather than eating and trying to swallow and digest food. I was becoming so scared to even put food into my mouth that I felt would block me up and make me more bloated and uncomfortable.

At the end of June I attended the hospital clinic to discuss the next step which was to have a scan done. It was here that it was confirmed I would undergo an internal and external ultrasound scan at the Hysteroscopy/Colposcopy Unit. It would be both an internal and external scan of my stomach area to get a better picture of what was happening.

A few days later and my friend Fiona was with me for support. Fiona drove up from Bournemouth. She had been through cancer herself and so empathised with what I was going through. Fi was diagnosed with a stage 3 Myxoid Fibrosarcoma. This cancer was in the skin on her back and Fi had undergone surgery in May 2013 at the hospital to have the cancer removed. I feel that it is not until you have experienced something like this yourself that you understand and appreciate what others before you have gone through. I know of many in my network, as well as those whose stories have come to light in the tabloids who have had their struggles with various cancers. I guess people with lots of money can pay to receive a wider spectrum of worldwide treatment and care. Nevertheless, if the cancer is caught too late then this still might not change their outcome. Cancer does not discriminate and can affect anyone, regardless of who they are.

It is strange how you know your own body and I kind of guessed it from the moment I first spoke with my GP nurse, yet I was still brushing it off as constipation. Now it was looking like something more serious and starting to head in the direction I didn't want it to go. Despite how much I didn't want it to be cancer related, I had a gut instinct that this was all going to lead to bad news. I tried to stay relaxed about it all and it helped having Fi there to support me.

It is all a bit of a waiting game with the various appointments and tests you must go through, which is probably one of the most frustrating things out of all of this. It is the wanting to know, and the time you spend stressing over what the outcomes could be. When you know something is not right, or you hurt so badly that you want the pain to go away, you want to be able to get the tests and results done like yesterday and move on to get it fixed. Unfortunately, most things don't happen that way and you must be patient and go through the process.

We were called through to a room by the oncologist, Dr Keay, who was the person carrying out the scan. She explained to me what the procedure would be and then asked me to step behind the curtain out of sight from Fiona and take off my clothing, put on a hospital gown and get comfortable on the bed.

An ultrasound scan (called a sonogram) is machinery that uses high frequency sound waves and is carried out to help doctors to gather information about your condition. This machinery creates images of part of the inside of your body and can show up anything looking abnormal.

Although I was given pre-scan criteria to read, Dr Keay ensured I understood everything that she was about to do and that I was happy with this procedure to take place using a small probe, which is what gives off the sound waves. These sound waves cannot be heard but they bounce off parts of your body and create echoes which are picked up by the probe and then create a moving image which is displayed on the monitor.

I was given the scans. For the external scan Dr Keay applied a lubricating gel to my skin. This makes the area smooth for a small handheld sensor to move freely over the area being examined. The gel felt slightly cold. Dr Keay then placed the sensor on my skin and slowly moved it around to examine my stomach area. This procedure can also examine the liver, kidneys and other organs in the tummy and pelvis, as well as other organs or tissues that can be assessed through the skin, such as muscles and joints.

The next stage was to carry out the internal ultrasound scan, also known as a transvaginal "through the vagina" ultrasound. This would entail a probe being inserted into my body to enable the doctor to look more closely at my internal organs such as my ovaries and womb. During the procedure I was made as comfortable as possible. A small ultrasound probe with a sterile cover, was gently passed into the vagina so that Dr Keay could capture images transmitted to a monitor. Internal examinations may cause some discomfort; however, I never felt any pain and it didn't take long to carry out.

Next on the hospital agenda was a specialist follow up appointment with a consultant and Macmillan nurse. The Princess Anne hospital is a place that specialise in gynaecological issues, breast mammograms and cancer consultations and is where many women go to give birth. This is the sister building across the road from the main General Hospital. Just knowing I was attending the Princess Anne kind of set the precedence for me for what was to come.

Chapter Three

Shit Happens

Friday, July 1st, 2016 - I had prepared for this and packed a notepad and pen with me. Mum offered to do the writing for me should I need it, whilst the doctor spoke to me.

The thing I hated most was the tension I could feel and the worry showing on my parents faces. No matter how much I could see they were being brave for me, I just knew how they must be feeling deep down inside. I was more worried about them and what they were about to find out as I know how devasting this forthcoming news could be. I was forty-seven, I was an adult, and I was independent; however, it doesn't take away the fact I was still their little girl in their eyes, and no one wants to hear bad news when it concerns your loved ones.

Together we walked in the main entrance and veered to our right to check in at the front desk.

"Hi, I'm Jacqueline Ridout, here to see Doctor Green."

The receptionist clicked on the computer screen to find my appointment, "all checked in for you. Please take a seat in the waiting area and you will be called through shortly."

We then turned around to find somewhere to sit in the large waiting room behind us. We must have each in our own minds had so much churning over and over that day. Knowing that at any minute my name would be called, and we would be walking into that room to hear my results. Sometimes we made small talk amongst ourselves to pass the time. I looked around the waiting area at the many people there, some who sat alone and those with their loved ones. I began wondering who out of these people were the victims and who were those there supporting the unfortunates.

"Jacqueline Ridout," a nurse by the name of Fiona introduced herself and called me through.

We followed her to a smaller waiting area adjacent to a corridor of doors.

"Hi Jacqueline, please take a seat here and this is where you will be called through to see Dr Green in her office."

I smiled and my parents and I took a seat. Eventually we were called in to the consultation room. It was a small square room with a bed along the back wall to our right as we walked in. We were asked to take a seat for which my dad perched on the bed against the back wall, and my mum and I sat on the chairs nearest the consultant's desk. I understand these people have a job to do and to have to give patients news, whether good or bad, must be the hardest thing in showing no emotion; however, the minute I stepped into that room I sensed it. I knew, and I braced myself for what was about to hit me. All I could think of was what my mum and dad were going through at this very moment and how they would react.

"Hello Jacqueline. My name is Claire Green and this is Fiona, one of our Macmillan team." And so, she began ...

"I have your CT scan results back and this does confirm that you have tumours on your ovaries and there are masses within your stomach. These are malignant tumours, so it is cancerous".

As she continued, my heart was pounding hard, and it felt like it would burst through my chest if it continued to beat any faster. It was as though I could loudly hear my blood pumping around my body, my blood pressure felt like it was suddenly rising, and my palms became sweaty, yet the only thing on my mind was my parents. I didn't think they would deal with this very well and this could be the one thing that could break them. Yes, I admit it, I was shocked, numb to the core and I felt sick. I had had a huge feeling this was what I was going to be told but it still did not prepare my mind that was now skidding out of control into a head on collision.

I sat there for some time listening intently to the words being spoken to me by the consultant. I was hearing it, but it was difficult to take it all in and to not focus too much on the negative side of it all. I hear people say so many times in conversations, "I heard the word cancer and all I could think about was dying". The word cancer seems to spell out DEATH to many and once they hear that word everything else falls on deaf ears.

Yes, I was shocked, and I felt an instant numbness and disbelief but, did I break down in a blubbering mess? ... No. Did I scream and shout? ... No. I just needed to know more, and I suddenly went from feeling completely numb to snapping out of it, and going into instant overdrive, batting back question after question that I needed answered.

"Can you tell me if the cancer is aggressive?"

Fiona the Macmillan nurse spoke, "yes, but we prefer to use the word advanced".

"Ok" I said, "what's the next step? is it curable? how long have I had this and how quickly do you feel this has grown?" I couldn't stop; it was question after question. My poor mum didn't use the notepad, not once, and I could see it was just too much information for both my parents to take in. I carefully took the note pad from my mum, and I started to jot down the answers as they were spoken to me. The consultant stopped and looked at me.

"Jacqueline, do you understand what I've just told you?"

"Yes, I do. I have advanced ovarian cancer; I have large tumours on my ovaries."

The consultant looked at me and asked, "have you anything else to say?"

I paused for a moment, looked around the room, then shrugged my shoulders and said, "shit happens". There was another pause as they all sat there looking at me as if waiting for me to continue. "I don't know what else to say to you but, shit happens."

I just felt numb at the thought of what rubbish would be going around in my mum and dad's minds. I had great concern for how my parents were feeling right at that moment. Everyone in the room fell silent. What else could I say? I have cancer. I needed to know what we were going to do to sort me out if anything?

Nobody wants to hear this news, and neither are they prepared for it. Nobody specifically saves for things like an unexpected illness. People save for holidays, weddings, cars, and the finer things in life for goodness' sake, not bloody cancer. Who wants to be dealt that hand in the game? However, with all these thoughts still racing around, I never thought 'why me'? Not once. It happens, and unfortunately, this time it was happening to me.

You can prepare all you want but when it comes to the day nothing pans out quite how you want it to. All of us are there trying to take in what is being said to us, dad in shock, mum in shock. Half the conversation goes over your head. You feel as if everything is suddenly moving on around you, but you have come to a silent standstill. You can see the consultant and nurse's lips moving but you do not hear or register everything that is being said to you. It is easy to just pick out certain words and if you aren't careful, it'll just be the negative things that you'll hear. I guess once you hear the word cancer, you associate it straight away with death.

For me I think the worst thing about cancer is not what it does to you, but what it does to those you love. My parents, although they had so much love for me yet so much worry at the same time, were more shocked at my determined response to it all, and my positive attitude to feel the need to find a way to fight it. I wanted to be strong for them. I knew we would have our moment, but I wanted to keep that bubbly, upbeat front I always have for their sakes because I knew they were crumbling inside. Their baby girl had just been told she has cancer. It could kill me. I might not have long to live. I might deteriorate in front of their very eyes. This is not how the story was meant to play out. I still had things I wanted to do. Or … I could keep focused and believe I could try to beat this invasion in my body.

I had so many emotions at that point, and I did think to myself *this is it, this is how I am going to die, and it is going to happen fast, this is my time to go*. I still felt my heart racing and I kept that thought for a moment longer. Then I just snapped out of it and thought, *no, this is not how it is meant to be, this cannot be the end for me*. I needed to find out more and ask more questions.

Harsh as it was, I wanted to know if I had minutes, days, weeks, months, or years left. I continued to ask question after question to get the answers I needed as to what we could do next? How could we fix this? What treatment would I receive? Would I lose my hair? (Not that it bothered me). Doctor Green confirmed that hair loss would happen. She mentioned a device called a cold cap that could possibly save my hair from falling out.

What else was there if the treatment failed? Was there a chance of survival and what chance did I have with regards to my results? The list of questions was endless. Between being told the answers and my research, I found out my cancer was at a stage 3 and my chances were 20% survival rate.

I was told I would have a biopsy to remove a sample of tissue from the tumours so they could be reviewed via a microscope and be tested to see what the cell type was, the most common type being a high grade serous, which is the most common type of epithelial ovarian cancers.

I was advised that some types of epithelial ovarian cancer respond better to chemotherapy treatment than others, and with mine being a stage 3 high grade serous cancer, it involves the ovaries or fallopian tubes. It can also spread to the peritoneum (stomach lining), outside of the pelvis and/or to lymph nodes in the retroperitoneum (lymph nodes along the major blood vessels, such as the aorta) behind the abdomen.

Benign or malignant, any sort of tumour can only cause problems, especially if it becomes more serious and starts to put pressure on nearby organs, which may weaken the overall bone structure, and can lead to broken bones or cause other problems.

Benign tumours may grow but cannot spread (metastasize) to anywhere else in the body. They stay localised in one area.

Malignant (cancerous) tumours which metastasize and spread to other parts of the body are known as secondary cancers. They can travel via the blood or the lymphatic system from the primary site where the cancer originally started.

Dr Green was amazing. She could see that I just wanted to know as much as possible and the questions did not stop coming. She freely answered as best she could to help me understand everything and give me as much helpful information as possible.

Because I had cancerous cells lasered from my cervix years ago, I wanted to know if this had anything to do with why the cancer was showing itself again in my body. I needed more information to know exactly what we were dealing with. I looked at Fiona and Dr Green, "can you tell me what stage this is at, because it feels like it will be high. When I had cancerous cells in my cervix years ago, I was told it was a SIN 3 and on the cusp of a SIN 3 to SIN 4. Is it that bad?"

Dr Green spoke, "it's stage 3 cancer. Due to it being ovarian and not being able to spot this so easily as some other cancers, it has grown quickly in size."

The nurse encouraged me to go sit on the bed behind where my parents were sitting. My dad was moved to one of the closer chairs with my mum where they continued talking to the consultant asking more and more questions. I could hear in their voices that they were just broken at this news. It was eating me up inside knowing their pain and heartbreak.

At this point the nurse closed the curtains around me, I began to silently cry on the bed. The nurse said, "this is why I brought you back here behind the curtain for a minute, so you can have your time and let it out".

I kept my voice low and explained how upset I was for my parents and how they must be feeling right now. I felt that they didn't need to be going through this rubbish at this time in their lives. They have both been my rocks, the people who brought me up and have given me a wonderful childhood and loved me endlessly. If this should get worse then the last thing that I wanted was them living out the rest of their lives looking after me. I should be looking after them at this time in their lives. The nurse, Fiona, gave me some reading to take home and the Macmillan team's contact details so I could call with any further questions I might have and for support moving forwards.

She then pulled the curtains back and we finished up our meeting with Doctor Green and made our way out of the hospital. My dad started to break down, my mum trying to be strong and hiding her feelings as usual, but I knew she was totally crushed. What mother wouldn't be? As we composed ourselves and walked through the waiting room, I felt as though all eyes were on us from the others sat there waiting in turn to be called in to hear their fate. I looked straight ahead as we walked through reception and continued our way out of the hospital. I do not really remember the journey home that day. I remember feeling numb, scared, worried, but I was also feeling hopeful and determined. I think we occasionally spoke of what we had been told and then the odd silence fell in between. We were all trying to hold it together during the journey home.

When we arrived home that day mum disappeared upstairs. Dad and I walked into their living room and dad broke down. We held each other, and we cried. I assured dad it would be okay, and we would do everything we could to fight this together. It broke my heart to think of mum upstairs as I knew she was trying to be brave for me and wanted to have her own time to deal with this news. Mum rarely gets upset in front of the family. All I wanted to do was to hold her and tell her everything would be alright, and it was crushing me that I couldn't, but I know she had to have her time and come back downstairs when she was ready.

Receiving this sort of news made me realise just how much I was worrying about what was going through their minds and how much I wanted to be brave for them and show them I wasn't going to let this beat me. I felt angry that cancer had decided to show itself and was affecting the two people I love most in the world. I felt like it was totally out of my control, but this made me want to fight all the way and to show my parents we were stronger than this and no matter what life threw at us, that love conquers all. Being hopeful is all that we could be at that time.

I hate cancer for breaking my parent's hearts and bringing them so much grief and devastation. I didn't like standing there watching their pain. I wasn't going to allow cancer to break us. It was not going to win and take away what we have.

I guess for me, the most frightening thing with all this was that it crept up on me. Some call it the silent and deadly killer; however, thinking about it, I don't believe this to be true.

Cancer can be multiplying within your body and grow to such an advance stage, but the fact is if I could have caught this sooner, it would not have reached the advanced stages and we could have dealt with this quickly. It must have been multiplying for quite some time, and due to the symptoms mirroring that of constipation, it was not picked up at my first GP visit.

These are the main symptoms of ovarian cancer, and the ones most charities speak of:

1: Bloating or a noticeable increase in your stomach size. For me, my stomach became so bloated that bruises became visible.
2: Feeling full quickly and having difficulty eating food.
3: Persistent stomach pains and twinges.
4: An urge to pee a lot more frequently than usual – like having a kind of wee infection sensation.
5: Bowel movements become less frequent, and you are constipated for more than 3 days.
6: Vaginal or back passage bleeding.

These are the key indicators for ovarian cancer, and I seriously urge women to act quickly and contact your GP to get checked out if you feel you have any of the main symptoms for this and you feel they are not going away.

If you have any initial concerns then start keeping a diary and write daily about your health and how you are feeling. Note what you ate and when, any activity you did, times of when you noticed things happening to your body, dates, and times when you spoke to your doctor about this, and if you are not satisfied with what you are being told, then do seek a second opinion before it becomes too late to deal with it.

I wanted to stay focused and believed I could do this. It was about researching and gathering the knowledge in which to help myself to stay fit and healthy and try to combat cancer.

I cannot keep urging people enough, if you are hesitating over something you feel is wrong with your body and you start to notice different or unusual changes, then go seek help from your GP and ask to have it checked out as soon as you start feeling this way. Do not leave it because if it is more serious it will not go away, it will still be there the day after and the day after that. This is your life, and this will affect the lives of your family members, your kids, your friends, your work life, your social life, everything. I think the quicker people nip such things in the bud the better all-round it can be. It may affect you short term if you must undergo treatment, but it will save you in the longer term if you take immediate action.

I know how detrimental this is now and I have lost many loved ones to different cancers, but I remember my friend Kerry losing her auntie Carol to ovarian cancer around 10 years ago. My cancer resembled similar patterns and went through the same stages Carol had gone through. Back then the medicine research was not as advanced as the drugs made available today. Through continued research and ongoing charity fundraising by many wonderful people, medicine has come a long way in the last 10 years or so. I feel if we had the medicines back then that we do now, more survivors would still be here in the world, on their personal journeys, and sharing their own success stories, including our lovely Carol.

I have spoken to people who question why the CA125 bloods cannot be done regularly in the same way as a cervical smear screening test is? I wish there were a test that could be introduced like that; one that could help doctors to detect ovarian cancer in the early stages before it becomes so advanced. We have come so far medically, that I pray in time such a test can be made available.

It was going to take us days to process and discuss all this information with each other, but I think this is where the therapy starts to kick in, by being open, talking it through and looking at how we will each deal with this together and try to overcome it.

I had to let my manager at work know what was going on. Once I had time to talk further with my parents and get it straight in my head, I called Jo to have a chat with her and explain what we had just been told. She was devastated to hear this news yet she kept calm and spoke clearly with her questions. Jo is particularly good at listening and knowing what to say in a variety of situations.

"Oh, dear Jackie, this isn't the news we were hoping for is it"?

We continued the conversation and Jo believed with a positive attitude I could tackle this head on. This was not the first time the company had been through something like this. Not long before I started my job, a young lad called Alex worked there in the Marketing team. His journey ended at a young age, and I heard that his manager, Katrina, who had been good work friends with Alex found this extremely hard, as did all the staff.

Alex had suffered for a short time with an aggressive cancer of the bile duct and not long before my joining, he passed away. One of his dreams was to see the Northern Lights. I found out he did get to make this journey to see them with his wife, Bryony, on their honeymoon. His passing affected his colleagues badly, so they took my situation very seriously from the moment I got my bad news.

Those individuals in my team who supported me through all this, they are the people who have kept me going daily, always checking on me to ensure how I was doing. They regularly spoke to me with such encouraging words that it pushed me to keep believing I could beat this. I love the fact that my work colleagues did not seem as if they were on the other side of the fence looking in at me showing pity; they were by my side every step of the way with me. They truly are remarkable people, and my manager Jo has been my work guardian angel from the moment I stepped foot across the threshold of that company.

Early July I decided to change my drinking habits. I have not been one for drinking lots of water in the past, so this was one thing I started to increase. I purchased decaffeinated coffee and tea bags. As the tumours were resting on my organs causing me to feel constipated, I knew I had to stay as hydrated as possible. I needed to do everything I could to ease the situation and help me to feel better.

I kept a food diary so I could look back to see if I had any issues with what I was eating. I was currently eating a lot less, due to my stomach feeling such discomfort and bloating.

Throughout the next couple of months I suffered with various ailments. Some days differed from others. I would suffer with leg pain, and a very taut feeling where my stomach was stretching, which was quite sore around my belly button. I experienced pains coming and going in my pelvic area and had bleeding and a discharge - I wore sanitary pads because of this - and going to toilet was difficult. My insides felt sore, and as though they were going to fall out. I have a high pain threshold, but this hurt and caused a lot of back passage bleeding. All this was down to the tumours resting on my organs and a build-up of fluid in my body, known as ascites. I continued to take remedies to help me find it easier to go to the toilet. Every night I would plump up my pillows and lay slightly upright on my back in bed with my hot water bottle as comfort. It was too painful to lay on my side and this was the only way I could get comfortable and manage to get some sleep.

My parents accompanied me to hospital for my first appointment for a CT scan, known as a Computed Lomography Body Scan. This was to be performed for my chest, abdomen, and pelvis with use of a contrast dye solution, and the scan would give the medical team a proper diagnosis of my condition. We arrived and checked in. Although I knew what was going to happen, I still felt a kind of trepidation about it. We were asked to wait in the waiting room, and I was given an oral contrast drink to sip over a 30-minute period to fill my bladder ready for the scan. This contrast dye would be able to highlight my blood vessels, organs and other structures and make it easier for the medical team to get a better picture of what was going on in my body. Next, I was asked to get gowned up in one of the side cubicles and then to sit on the seats just outside the scanning room. There I was, sat ready and waiting, gowned up with a belly full of contrast. A few minutes passed and then the radiographer reappeared.

"Jacqueline, would you like to come on through."

I was then taken through to a large bright room, all white and clinical smelling. There was a big circular scanning machine situated in the middle of the room with a bed which glided through the machine once it started. To the left was a glass panelled wall, and the room was similar but on a larger scale to that of an X-Ray room. I was asked to lay down on the bed and then a canula was put into my arm.

"We're going to flush the vein through with saline to check all is working okay before we start."

The staff explained what was going to happen so I was fully aware, and that the CT scan would take 6 X-rays as a 3-dimensional picture of my abdomen area. Firstly, the bed moved through the circular shaped CT scanning machine and did a cycle with an injection of the dye. As the CT scanner whirled around doing its thing, the noise sounded like a washing machine on a fast spin. Next a pre-recorded voice said, "breathe in and hold", I did so, it then it said, "breathe out".

Then for the next scans, the dye was to be injected into my arm, and this would help to show a clearer picture of my insides. The radiographer told me to tell them if I felt my skin become very irritated or sting, and then he went behind the glass panel and the scanning process started again. The scanning bed moved through the machine, and I could feel the dye entering my arm.

The dye gave me quite a warm feeling as it passed through my veins. It was a feeling like you get after rubbing deep heat on your skin. No sooner had it entered my body, than I felt it travelling quickly, in seconds, from my arm to my stomach and then straight to my legs. The warm rushing sensation of the dye made me feel as if I was wetting myself.

For some reason, I could not stop shaking. Not sure why as I felt okay. Just think my nerves got the better of me, probably as this was the first time I had something like this done. The staff in the room made me feel comfortable; they were literally holding my hand and making general chit chat as they had noticed me shaking so much. What was all the fuss about? It was done within minutes, no pain, just me on a moving table, passing back and forth through the large circular whirring machine. I felt as if I was in some sort of sci-fi movie and Han Solo was about to walk in to save me ... wishful thinking that one!

My follow up meeting was held with Dr Keay and it was confirmed that I had aggressive ovarian cancer. Dr Keay told me I had masses in my stomach area and there were tumours on each ovary seven centimetres long. This clarified my earlier assumption as being spot on and she agreed that the tumours were the size of tennis balls. Dr Keay told me that I still needed to have the biopsy on Wednesday, so we could determine exactly what we were dealing with. *Crikey*, I thought. "How many more experiments are they going to perform on me until they get to the core of it?"

This was so not great news, I had mixed emotions right then, feeling very scared. I still had this need to stay positive and brave for my parents and my loved ones. I was worrying about the time I would need off work, I felt deflated, I wanted to fight this, I was too young to have this and most of all how long did I have left on this earth?!

Reality was beginning to sink in and I felt helpless for my parents, I can't die - how would they cope? I refused to allow this disgusting disease to invade my body any further, I wanted rid, and I chose to fight. So many thoughts and feelings ran through my confused little head right then. My feelings were changing from emotional worry to a positive 'I can beat this' attitude. The consultant thought I would have 6 chemotherapy cycles in total. Possibly looking at 3 chemo and then a full hysterectomy operation (depending on how much the chemo shrunk the cancer) and then another 3 treatments after the operation.

I drew a diagram to show the doctor my uterus and I had Dr Keay draw on the diagram where the tumours and the seedlings were.

I wanted to know where the hard lumps were situated and how many? Were they in the peritoneum and omentum, and would this be taken away with chemo or surgery? Was it top, bottom, all around the stomach? When the doctor said advanced, did she mean it had spread quickly locally or was it widespread and so aggressive that it was possibly too late? Dr Keay described some of the stages of cancer to me from 1b being cancer in both ovaries to 1c having cancer in both ovaries with cells leaking to the abdomen/pelvic area.

Dr Keay explained that the CA125 blood tests are done to check for raised levels of protein, as this shows any activity happening within my body. She said I am at a stage 3, and in my case, when it spread outside the ovary, it had stayed in the abdominal cavity, so it had "locally spread".

I wanted to know everything. Why was the cancer likely to re-occur? What was the ratio for secondary cancer? If it came back, where would it be likely to appear? Is this when they would look to put me on the Avastin maintenance drugs to prolong my life and keep the cancer controlled to an area? Could I have radiotherapy if the chemotherapy didn't work? What was my life expectancy? Would I benefit from treatment? I mean, they told me it was a 20% cure rate, right? Was I understanding all this correctly? This scared me into thinking I didn't have much of a chance of survival. Had it spread to my lymph nodes? My head was full of so many questions and my feelings keep shifting.

Although the doctors treat many people for the same type of cancer, I had to keep reminding myself that we are each in this world quite different, and the doctors can only give me guidance based on the type of cancer and my personal situation. I see it that they were just as much in the dark and were doing their best to help me to survive. They could treat someone remarkably like me, but the outcome could still be different.

Dr Keay advised the scan was not showing any insignificantly enlarged abdominal or pelvic lymph nodes; however, there was a small volume of asities (fluid) present.

I understood it that when a cancer is so advanced, it is possibly not something that is curable. Statistically ovarian cancer is likely to come back and the Macmillan nurses and gynae medical team were going all out to try to help me to maintain this. Macmillan understood I wanted to improve my quality of life and outcomes. I was advised to eat a well-balanced low fibre diet, and Dr Keay advised by eating low fibre for now it should help the stomach pressure I was currently feeling.

"What if the cancer isn't killed off? I know from knowledge of other past experiences in life that cancer seedlings can be so microscopic, they sprinkle off like when you blow on a dandelion, and these can lay dormant and grow back over time." I paused and then continued, "there have been cases where a person's cancer doesn't show again, so is this because the microscopic seedlings were caught and killed off? Is it a case of the longer the cancer stays away, the less aggressively it is growing and can be controlled?"

Dr Keay spoke, "if it comes back within 6 months, a fast return such as this is very advanced. If the cancer doesn't return for around 2 years then this is a slower growing cancer, however the disease can mutate and change."

I then drew another diagram and asked Dr. Keay to show me where within the peritoneum and lymph nodes, these masses (tumours) were.

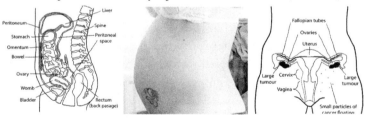

I went with the hospital advice and with what I felt comfortable with when researching. I found the best websites to research on are the charity websites such as Macmillan, Cancer Research, Target Ovarian Cancer, Ovacom, Tenovus Cancer Care, Jane Scarth, Penny Brohn – the list goes on, and once you contact one charity, or hear of charities through hospital discussions, it will open a whole new world of help and information. The charities will give you details or put you in touch with any others they feel would be of help to you. All I can say is that the support network out there is awesome once you start asking for help.

I feel it is safer to stick to just the cancer charity websites as they have good informative criteria to read through and understand. Whereas researching the web in any available content can be dangerous. You can easily find conflicting information which can scare the hell out of you as you could be reading about a person's condition which sounds like your own, but their outcome could differ completely to how yours will be and Dr. Google is NOT the way forward.

After this meeting I decided to change up a gear with my diet and look to boost my intake of more good foods to help with my recovery. I felt I needed to do more to help my body stay strong and healthy. I set to work and with some pre-planning and making a change to my food shopping list for cancer fighting ingredients, I began my quest.

I am not one for eating much fruit; so I chose to introduce more of this to my diet. To ensure I got the goodness into my body daily I decided to juice the fruit up into smoothie form; that way I would be more likely to incorporate this into my daily routine as I could carry this on the go when needed.

I went straight out and purchased myself a smoothie machine, did a large shop for ingredients, and whizz away I did! Most of my smoothies consisted of a large variety of fruits, with banana-based options or dark berries. I tested and tried many concoctions, some of which tasted a bit too sweet, yet I kept this up to get as much goodness into my body as I could.

As with all research you need to be careful and along the way I read up on other articles that popped up. Certain foods such as red meats are not great for the digestive or bowel system for many people, so having my ovarian issues, I also decided to cut out red meat and stick to chicken, fish, vegetables, and salad. As a treat I would occasionally have red meat and other naughty foods when going out to dinner that I purposely did not stock at home, thus doing away with the temptation! If I know there is nothing naughty sitting in my cupboards, then I can't eat rubbish. I felt that taking away the temptation was a good move to make sure I just ate the right foods to condition myself and my body

My diet has generally been quite a healthy one, and yet now I introduced more vegetables to my plate, the usual things you know you should bulk out your dinner plate with, but rarely do. I believe these changes I was consciously making was helping me to make a big difference to my body and well-being.

Throughout the lead up to all of this, my time was spent researching between Dr Green's clinics. I posed more and more questions about food and highlighted to the best of my beliefs about sugar and how harmful it is to our bodies. The various people I spoke with listened to me and advised me that I should just eat what I want and if I wanted to eat well then, I should still have a bit of naughty food in my diet. People could see how much I wanted to find a way to fight this and were taking on board the fact that I was finding out lots of information. The medical staff said I could drink as much prosecco as I wanted, yet I laughed this off as a bit of a joke between us, nurses trying to lighten the mood of a bad situation and making me see I could still live my life normally.

I guess from a medical perspective they couldn't really comment but only encourage me to eat a good balanced diet. Maybe medically they cannot answer dietary questions like this. After all, their forte is ovarian cancer, not bloody master chef!

There is so much useful information out there on the web and in books for a varied number of diets. My diet needed to consist of things that could help me to build up my white cells and keep me strong enough so I'd be ready for the treatment three weeks later.

I try to alternate my food shopping to give me a change as well as variety to keep my interest up and keep my body fighting. These are just a few of the things I eat regularly in my meals and breakfasts to ensure I am getting a good intake of vitamins and minerals and fatty acids. Organic foods and naturally reared foods are best as most are grown/reared without the use of pesticides, hormones, and other chemicals. Bright coloured vegetables such as food like red bell peppers, spinach, kale, tomatoes, oranges, watermelon, sweet potatoes are all carotenoid foods and they act as antioxidants, anti-inflammatory and they are good for the immune system.

Various red fruits, dark leafy greens, avocado, broccoli, poultry - I like chicken noodle soup with garlic as it is good for you if you make it from scratch with chicken broth, plain full fat yoghurt to dollop on my low sugar cereal. I never choose low fat products as they are much higher in sugar. I make my cereal using dark berries, coconut flakes, cinnamon oats, and a variety of nuts, as nuts contain zinc, omega 3, fatty acids and Vit E antioxidants.

Mushrooms have great anti-tumour/anti-bacterial benefits for your body, as does garlic, matcha tea and turmeric. The best mushrooms for a cancer patient to eat are the oriental kind such as shiitake or reishi.

I make regular use of spices, herbs and black pepper and I drink green tea (adding ginger and lemon) and Rooibos tea for antioxidant benefits.

Oily fish (omega 3), shellfish (zinc) which is good for strengthening the immune system. Zinc will help to increase your white blood cells and the T Cells which fight infection.

With my research I found some conflicting dietary information on the web. I read that fruit seeds can cause constipation, and to juice rather than blend, avoiding fruit skins and pulps. Also, there was advice on taking care which fruits you juice together due to the amount of sugar being processed together in one smoothie.

This again is why I believe sugar feeds cancer, so I wanted to know if keeping as much sugar out of my diet as possible would help me to stay cancer free and live a healthier and longer life? I touch more on sugar and foods later in this book.

Still, in the back of my mind I began to wonder if I was doing the right thing. Maybe everyone was telling me they thought I should just try and lead as normal a life as possible without going too far off the Richter scale with my healthy eating concoctions because they knew something I didn't. Were they just trying to tell me in a roundabout way to live my life each day as if it was my last? They were trying to lighten the blow for me, right? Maybe I didn't really have a chance at even trying new things to beat this? Just maybe the truth was I was going to die?!!

Smack, bang, wallop! Right there at that moment the actual thought of death presented itself to me like the bright flashing lights of Vegas. *Crikey, is this what they are trying to tell me?* I sat in my clinic meeting projecting my usual sunshine into the room whilst listening to my doctor's answers to things I had asked, yet inside I had these other questions beginning to dart around my mind, back and forth, up and down, like a pinball machine. My focus was still there in the room but the thought of death lingered just there in the background, never too far away at this point.

That's the thing. You can hear something, or not hear what you want to hear, and you can take it completely out of context to how it is being explained to you. You can get something in your head that will start to eat away at you, and you can end up thinking the worst before you've even got started. It's times like this that I wish I had a crystal ball, that bit of insight before the event takes place … now that is one hell of a superpower to wish for! It's the not knowing that scares people about cancer, and probably why straight away people associate this with death, as death is the unknown to us all. I quickly reined my thoughts back in to a better way of thinking, *stay positive, do not give up now, you've still got a chance.* These were the thoughts that were keeping me sane and giving me the willpower to want to do something about this.

The forthcoming treatment process was explained to me, so I knew what to expect. Firstly, I would be having approximately 6 chemo-therapy treatments. In week 1 of each treatment, I could expect side effects during this period where my joints would feel achy, and within approximately 3 to 4 days the sickness and tiredness would kick in. I was told I might also feel a slight numb, tingling sensation to my skin, as treatment can affect the nerves.

Once into the second week, I would still feel tired, and this is where my immune system would be at its lowest. My white blood counts would drop down to rock bottom, and this is when I would be most at risk of infection and would need to be careful around people with colds.

Week 3 is when I would start to notice the hair loss.

My body would certainly need the fluid intake to prevent dehydration so the main thing was to ensure I regularly drank enough water – another thing I have never been great at doing. However, moving forwards I would do whatever was needed to keep my body in good shape to combat what it would be going through. All this would probably help me to combat the sickness side of things, too.

The discussion arose again of the option of me wearing a cold cap during my treatment. This can be an extremely uncomfortable thing to go through as it gives you an achy, brain freeze like feeling to your head. I can certainly remember the painful brain-freeze sensation I used to get as a child from drinking back slush puppies too fast or eating ice-cream, and it would give me that sharp cold feeling hitting me right in my forehead. I imagined this could only be 10 times worse!

The doctor proceeded to explain that due to my thick, full, long curly hair, the type of cancer I had, along with the harsh cocktail of chemotherapy drugs I would have to endure, it was likely the cold cap would struggle to work on me, and I was highly likely to lose most of my hair, if not all of it, anyway.

I totally understand why many women would probably take that chance and choose to go through with it. It is an important part of your femininity disappearing, part of your looks changing, the fact of being a woman and going completely bald. I get it. But for me, if there was nothing to show at the end of it, then what was the point?

There was no way I was even contemplating putting myself through that torture if I was going to be zapped with harsh chemotherapy and experience the whole time sat with complete brain freeze for a "maybe" outcome.

Straight away I refused to waste the hospitals and my time using one of these as I would be going through enough trauma, without the added pain of wearing something that wasn't going to save my long curly locks anyway. Plus, this could be going to good use helping another cancer patient who did have the need for it and the knowledge that this cap would save their hair. Having no hair at the end of all this was not the issue … having my life was.

Dr Green advised I would meet the surgeon, Mr Hadwin, at my pre-op assessment appointment on Friday October 21ˢᵗ.

"Jackie, at this meeting you will have the chance to ask further questions with the surgeon and he will discuss the operation procedure with you. It will be a debulking operation of your ovaries, tubes, cervix, and part of the stomach omentum. Your cervix will be rebuilt up. *Gosh*, I thought. *They can rebuild me, just like the bionic woman.*

I sat, I thought, and yep, I just had to question it … "will my op affect my sex drive or how sex can feel to me?"

"Sometimes this can change for a person, and you can expect possible dryness."

We discussed and agreed I should come off the pill as I did not have a man in my life, and I was having everything removed.

"I've heard through others that sometimes staples are used during surgery. Will I be stitched or stapled?"

"Jackie, this will depend on what the surgeon's usual closure is."

"Will there be much post-bleeding and discharge, and will I need to take my own sanitary pads to hospital?"

"Yes, you will need these; they aren't always necessary but better to be prepared." "Do I get anything to use from the NHS such as a walking stick?"

"No, you won't need it, the hospital will ensure they have you up and walking about quite quickly".

Questions, questions, questions – those poor nurses were certainly kept entertained during my visits.

Still "chewing" over the previous food conversations I had had in my clinics, I started thinking about my low white blood count. If my white blood count was low, then how could I raise this?

In brief: our bone marrow is a sponge-like tissue, and within the centre of our bones is where our platelets, red and white blood cells are made. Our blood cells replace themselves with new cells every so often; however, such things as having chemotherapy or radiotherapy treatment can affect the bone marrow and prevent it making enough white blood cells. Therefore, every second week of my treatment would be when my immune system would be at its lowest and I would be more susceptible to infection.

I feel it can be dangerous to research too many different websites and blogs as the information can start to get conflicting. These are the opinions of others for what they believe works, and this will not always be correct for your own personal diagnosis. It can scare the living daylights out of you if you start believing everything you read. What might be the case for one person is NOT the case for the next. Even if a person were to have the same cancer as someone else, they still could receive a different cocktail of chemotherapy depending on their body type, how aggressive the cancer is, etc. We are all different and in each person's case, we can have allergies and be susceptible to different things such as foods, treatments and the drugs given.

I do also strongly believe in trying to take the positives from any situation and doing what you can to help yourself. My research for my diagnosis to help my body is just my opinion and approach on how I chose to deal with this obstruction in my life. No one was certain how long I was going to live or if they could help with treatment. All I know was once diagnosed, the hospital wanted to do all they could to help me, and I believed in them and that my story was not ready to end just yet. I was determined to fight this all the way and stay as positive as possible and see this through. I admit I was scared but I was not ready to give up and I was determined to do all that I could to stay strong and be well again.

I met up with a gang of friends one evening for dinner in the shell of our friend's house that was being built. We sat eating fish and chips and catching up. Lynne noticed how restrained my mood was compared to usual and guessed that something was wrong. I normally tend to wear my heart on my sleeve; however, I thought I was hiding my feelings quite well up until she asked me if I was okay. I mentioned my stomach and that I was having further tests done. I didn't stay on this conversation for too long as I wanted to try and enjoy the evening with everyone. Lynne, although she did not show any great concern outwardly to me at the time, admitted much later that she was worried about me on that night.

Chapter Four

Biopsy

The morning of July 20th had arrived, and I was in the Surgical Day Unit at 07:00 sharp for a 07:30 image guided biopsy. I prepped my body a couple of days prior to this appointment washing with a hospital hibiscrub, an antimicrobial cleanser. This helps patients having any kind of operation to manage infections pre and post operation. Though you only need to use it two days before, being a bit of a safety girl, I chose to do this for approximately 4 days before I was admitted being sure of preventing possible infection. My parents came in to sit with me after I was gowned up and then put on a bed. We sat chatting for a bit and then two porters arrived at my bedside to take me to another area of the hospital to have my biopsy. As they wheeled me away on the hospital bed, my parents watched on as we disappeared down the corridor and out of sight. I gave them a smile, they smiled back, but again I could tell the agony they were both going through.

I am not going to lie, I had two painful experiences during the whole time of my illness, and the biopsy was one of them. The doctors explained as to what was going to happen and that they would put the needle into my stomach and move it around to find the tumours on my ovaries. They would then pierce from inside this to grab a tiny amount of tissue with what looked like a tiny claw on the end of the needle. This would need to be done three times. I lay there, and they started the machine ready for procedure.

"Okay Jacqueline, just try to relax, we're going to start".

The doctor began the process whilst the male nurse was busying about in the room helping her. The needle was carefully put into my stomach. There was some moving about, and the doctor was looking at the computer screen to find the tumours.

"Okay Jacqueline", she said calmly, "I'm ready to go in to take the first one".

Then suddenly out of nowhere, I experienced the most excruciating pain I have ever felt in my life. I could not believe what the hell I was experiencing. The tiny claw inside the needle quickly injected into my body and grabbed some tissue from one of the tumours. My body literally convulsed at what seemed like inches to me, right off the bed, as though I had been given a full pulse of a defibrillator machine. I felt my body shaking so hard and it wouldn't stop. This certainly was NOT what I was expecting.

The nurse shot swiftly around to my bedside to comfort me, and he held my hand ready for the next one. *Seriously*, I thought, *do I really have to go through this, two more times?* I gripped onto the poor bloke's hand as if I was on a white-knuckle ride.

As the procedure continued, I was dreading each punch to the stomach, each part of my microscopic size of flesh being ripped from the tumours in my stomach. I know it was a small price to pay to help me get better, but it was a bloody painful one! Unfortunately for me, the doctor informed me she was taking a fourth biopsy to ensure they had taken enough tissue to analyse. I lay there trying to think positively but also just wanting it to all be over.

The days between tests and treatments varied, from going to watch my friend's son's football tournament and visiting my cousin's new-born baby, these being good days, to then being in much pain on the bad days at home with a very sore belly button area and more fluid and bleeding occurring.

Night times I was experiencing high temperatures and, in bed, with aching legs and back. At these times I found your mind is more likely to work overtime, and I had a sense of feeling alone and very scared.

The butterflies in the stomach would come back. I did not want this cancer invading my body!

Over a week later I was back at the hospital. After playing the waiting game for so long, in-between having my many tests, and being prodded and poked about like a specimen, I was finally going to get my biopsy results. We knew it was cancer anyway, but this would be the green light to get cracking on with it.

The main building is normally the go to place for the majority of tests, bloods, treatment, etc, whereas, when you are attending an appointment at the Princess Anne, then you know you are going to get told something not good.

My appointment was for midday. I had been staying with my parents for the ten days since the biopsy, to recuperate. On our way to hospital, we were keeping the conversation light-hearted. I love my parents more than life itself, and I knew they were feeling just the same as me.

"Hey mum, you guys will be glad when I go home tomorrow."

Mum looked back at me in the car and smiled, "I'm going to bill you for the use of the electric for all the smoothies you've been making, my dear!". We laughed.

The journey to the hospital was nearly at its end, and I was still jotting questions down ready to ask the consultant. I was apprehensive but still determined. I knew I could do this.

The biopsy results confirmed everything the doctors had said previously – I had Stage 3 Advanced Ovarian cancer. We sat and discussed it, and I posed various questions again. Once we finished up, my parents and I went for a coffee together and then I had to think about how I would broadcast this kind of news to individuals in my family - one of the most upsetting and terrifying things I had to face.

My parents asked me how I wanted to play this? After much debating and talking about it, I thought it best that it came from me so that I could explain the situation over the phone to each household. This way I could get it off my chest and if they had questions, I could answer them. I didn't want to shy away from this or for people to shy away from asking me things. I wanted to be open about this and felt it would be a way of releasing any stress that might be building up inside if I talked about it freely.

This was not an easy decision to make. My family are my world and I know how much it upsets me when I hear their bad news. It was a job that had to be done and the sooner I got settled back home, the sooner I could start this awful process of picking up the phone and dialling each number and just telling it straight, how it was and to ensure they understood that I was determined to stand up to cancer and not give in easily.

My worry was how they would each react and how this would make them feel due to the fact we had all been here many times before with other family members. They would each understand to a certain extent because of the nightmares they had previously faced with cancer.

Number one on my list was Tony, my brother. After this I started to make the rounds with the family calls. I took a deep breath, looked at my mobile and then began dialling. One after the other, call after call, it got slightly easier for me, although it still was not a nice thing to have to do.

It became quite draining receiving the many calls and texts from people that day. It was not the first time in our family that we had had to face cancer, but at least it was out there now. The worst part was done. All my loved ones knew.

It was the first day of August and I was feeling emotional. I had never thought *why me*, it never even entered my mind. Some people I have spoken to have said "you must have thought, why me?" but, no, I never did. Obviously, I never wanted to end up with anything like this, but I had. I strongly believe that it is how you deal with it that can help in making a difference. It can seem easy to feel like giving up straight away, but I feel unless you try, then you will never know. I have heard of stories of survivors that were told they had little time or there was nothing more that could be done for them, yet they are here today.

The following day I was meeting up with my friend's mum, Hilary, for lunch. Hilary recommended a place called Jane Scarth which is a cancer charity in Romsey close to my job. We decided to go there together so that Hilary could introduce me to the place, and I could talk to someone about what they do.

The staff are so helpful, and they have a vast range of leaflets about Macmillan and other cancer charity organisations. Jane Scarth can only do what they do because of the generosity of the public through donations or fundraising events. It is a place of calm, where you are greeted with a friendly welcome and a nice cuppa. They are there for you to listen, advise and they are people who do empathise and understand, especially as some themselves have been affected by cancer. They have various rooms where you can have counselling or book free therapeutic treatments to help you whilst you are on your cancer journey, and thereafter if needed.

I have tried various things since starting my journey and still attend occasionally when I have a bad day, or I feel I need a completely different face to speak to rather than to someone who is emotionally attached to me.

Jane Scarth, like the hospital Macmillan Centre, is a place that makes me take a step back, stop and breathe for a moment and think about me, no one else, just me. They have certainly helped me to rid my emotional build up and do good to my body and mind with the various treatments, exercises, and coffee breaks I have there.

Hilary was diagnosed with breast cancer in March 2006, just before her birthday. She had lost her hair through treatment. In the June of 2006, it was the hottest day of the year and Hilary's son Stu was getting married. Hilary wore a wig that day and how she got through it is beyond me. She was still having chemotherapy and radiotherapy treatment, which continued until December 2006.

Hilary inspired me so much because she still found the strength and confidence to wake up, get herself ready and attend her son's big day. I love her for her courage and the fact she researches a lot of things from foods to cosmetics, to find natural remedies and ways to help her combat cancer and stay cancer free.

Around this time, I was still suffering badly with the constipation. I had been trying all sorts from prune juice, hot water bottle, peppermint tea, increasing my water intake, suppositories, etc. Going to the toilet was an effort but I persisted in trying things to make me feel a bit more comfortable.

The day after I met with Hilary, was spent with my friend, Jo, her husband Matt, and my little goddaughter Phoebe. They had been over during the afternoon with a few food items for me and they stayed at my flat until early evening. Jo was at that time on a walking stick due to various issues of her own and was awaiting an operation to fit a pelvic plate, but as always, she was putting others before herself.

I was resting on my bed the whole time they were with me. Both my right leg and my back were aching, and my stomach was very sore to the touch and felt tight. When I got up to go to the toilet there was a yellowish fluid coming from my back passage, which was now another worry, in fact a big worry for me. It was starting to get late, so they got up to go home. We said our goodbyes and walked to the front door. Jo's last words to me were, "please call me if you get in any more pain and I will come back and get you to hospital if need be".

As I got settled back into bed for the night, I was hoping the pain would subside, but it was becoming more and more unbearable. For some time I was tossing and turning to try to get in a comfortable position. I used pillows to wrap my leg round, then tried laying on my back, and again on my side. I couldn't sleep, and I started to think bad things and worry that if something inside my stomach might rupture that I could experience a bad infection or organ failure, or have a reflux in my sleep and choke, or die and no one would know. I burst into tears with fear and laid for some time holding my stomach crying and shaking with fright. Never have I ever felt anything like the fear that was in me that night; like I was going to die if I did not act on it soon. Eventually I pulled myself together, sat up slowly, dried my eyes and thought about what I needed to do.

These horrid feelings and this uncomfortableness went on for some time, I was in so much pain and I knew it would only get worse, so I surrendered to the fact I needed to contact Jo and get to that hospital pronto. The time was around 21:50 so I called the weekend emergency doctor. He asked me quite a few questions to determine how bad he thought I was, and then he made the decision for me to get into hospital and he would organise to have a bed ready for my arrival.

"Do you have someone who can bring you in tonight Jacqueline?"

"Yes I do. I'll make the call to my friend now and we can get back to you within around half an hour or so. She will need to drive to pick me up and then we'll be on our way." We finished our conversation.

I hesitated about making that call and worry Jo further. Jo wasted no time, and she was in her car and back at my flat within fifteen minutes of my call. She called my mobile once she arrived outside and I slowly made my way out to her car to make our way to the hospital. As we walked up to the ward reception desk a nurse was there ready to talk to us. She confirmed they had a bed made up ready for me for the night and she took Jo and I to where I would be staying.

They gave me various meds and a stomach injection, then also took my bloods and blood pressure. Next I was asked to try suppositories to see if that might help but, still nothing was happening. Jo sat with me until the early hours of the morning. At around 02.30 I turned to Jo and asked her to go home as I was here for the duration and was being looked after.

"Okay," Jo said, "only if you are absolutely sure".

"Yes honey, there's no point in you staying here any longer, otherwise you're going to be knackered. Go home to Matt and Phoebe."

Jo looked at me, "alright, I'm just going to the toilet and then I'll head on home, and you can try to get some sleep". As Jo got up and started hobbling on her walking stick out to the hospital toilets, I watched her disappear out of sight, then I lay there on the bed thinking about what this amazing person had just done for me.

Jo went out of her way, even though she couldn't walk properly and was in her own pain, she still came back to get me and bring me here to get the help I needed. At that point I don't quite know what happened, but my emotions took over and I lay there quietly sobbing into my pillow. I felt like I couldn't stop but I knew I had to get myself together before Jo returned to say goodnight. The last thing I wanted was for her to come back and see me in a state. I didn't want her worrying and I needed her to get to her car and back home safely. Jo returned, we chatted for a bit. Jo wanted to sort a few things out with me before returning home … "and then when I get up tomorrow, I'll contact your parents to explain what's happened and they can come here to be with you".

When Jo eventually left, I tried to get myself comfortable. I felt so much discomfort and tightness. My stomach felt solid to touch, and I lay awake for what seemed like an exceptionally long time. I don't remember exactly when I drifted off, but I did manage to catch some sleep that night.

Morning came and I awoke still in pain. There was more bleeding and fluid seeping out below. My stomach looked as if at any moment Alien would come bursting out at the seams in good old blood-splattering fashion. To be honest, at that moment I would have welcomed that just to stop the agonising pain I was in and alleviate this tautness and pressure. At 08.10 the nurse advised me that they would give it two more hours and if nothing was moving, then they would look to give me an enema to try to help move things along. At around 09:00 a male nurse popped in to talk with me.

"Good morning, Jacqueline. How are we doing today?"

He explained he was there to assess me and then he began asking a few questions. My temperature and blood pressure were taken, and we chatted some more.

"We're going to leave you until around 10.30/11:00 and if nothing has happened by then, we'll look at giving you an enema." I nodded and I felt really fed up with it all.

"Jacqueline, are you happy for me to give the enema or would you rather a female nurse did this for you?" At this point I really didn't care I just wanted the pain to disappear and for my stomach to feel a bit normal again.

Without thinking I looked at the male nurse and said, "Yes, I am happy for you to stick it up me".

The moment those words left my mouth I wanted the ground to swallow me up immediately. My brain does not always engage with my mouth before I speak, and I have been known many a time to crack out some good one-liners or say things that get me into trouble. He was very professional and just smiled then departed from the ward to get prepped. I lay there feeling a little hot under the collar thinking *oh gosh, my big brainless mouth. Why?* This procedure is not a painful thing to have done but it's not a nice thing to experience. It took a while for things to happen and although it wasn't a full-blown showstopper, as soon as my body surrendered, they gave me the green light, got the paperwork to discharge me and that was that. Phew! Hallelujah!

A few more days passed, and Fiona and Jacquie came to see me at my flat. The swelling of my stomach had reached my boobs and I was looking more like humpty dumpty than a size eight. This worried me a lot as I had expected a fast reaction once I had had the enema. I constantly drank lots of water to flush through my body, although I still felt much pain. I guess water would only do better than harm and would keep me well hydrated and things shifting slightly. We arranged to meet for lunch the following day with Serena and Karen, at a coastal restaurant called Banana Wharf in Hamble marina. The marina is set in the heart of the south coast and many visitors who descend upon Hamble consist of sailing and racing enthusiasts. There is always a great atmosphere here and it was lovely to spend time with them all, even though we all knew how serious this was becoming. As I was eating my food, I realised my throat was feeling uncomfortable when swallowing and my chest hurt. It felt like a weighted down aching kind of feeling. I said nothing and continued to enjoy the moment with my friends. As I watched them talking and laughing, I sat feeling conscious this could be the last time, if things didn't work out for me, that I'd not get the chance to do anything like this with them again.

That evening I sat thinking for a while about everything that was happening to me, and I began to think about my friend in America, Jeni. I decided to call her for a chat. Jeni is like a sister to me and as usual we talked for an exceptionally long time. Although distance is between us, it seems no object when you can just pick up the phone and make a video call these days.

I love America, I love the people, I love the good vibes it gives me as well as the sunshine, and Jeni certainly brings a great deal of that into my life. I call Jeni's family my second family because that is what they have been to me from the moment I first met them. Our friendship began at the age of thirteen from an ad placed in a teen magazine. My school friend initiated it, and within a few weeks the Duran Duran fans of Southampton, England were writing to our pen-pals, the Duran Duran fans of Phoenix, Arizona. Since we put pen to paper all those years ago, Jeni and I are the only ones who stayed in contact, and we have become great friends over the years with a few visits back and forth to each other. The last time I set foot on American soil was back in 2008. The only thing I dislike about the distance is that it has become longer between our visits to each other over the years, and sometimes all you really want to do is reach out and give each other a hug.

Jeni lost her dad, Bill, to cancer. He had been sick for a while and even though it was expected, it hit hard with his passing. Both he and his wife Shirley were amazing people and on my first trip to them at eighteen, they went all out to take me to various places. We all travelled in an RV across Arizona for a few days, stopping in Sedona, Vegas, the Grand Canyon, LA and back to Phoenix. I took in the whole American adventure and instantly fell in love with the place and the people.

When Jeni and I get on the phone we always have so much to catch up on and so we both talk for England (and America!). I love Jeni's positive, laid-back attitude and the fact she speaks many words of wisdom to me, throwing in her good sense of humour along the way. I call her my sister across the pond. We live so far apart yet we feel so close. She should have used her life skills and studies to become a shrink. Whenever we get into deep conversation Jeni finds the solution.

As soon as our call was over, I sat on my bed and the flood gates opened. I could not control the tears and I cried for around ten minutes. I couldn't stop my emotions spilling over, or the hurt I was feeling about my situation and the people in my life it was also affecting. Was this it for me? Would it stop me doing what I love, my job and livelihood, my social circles, my photography? Was this how my life was going to be or end? Would it be a turning of tables with my parents having to take care of me instead of me taking care of them? And worse still, would they and my brother have to watch me gradually deteriorate and die? Was I ever going to be well enough to have nice holidays? Would I ever get the chance to go back and do another American road trip to see Jeni and her family? Would I be around to watch our ever-growing family of cousins and still enjoy life with them? And what about my never-ending gigs and festivals? Or was I going to be forever confined indoors? My mind was racing, and I sat pondering the many scenarios in my head.

It can't be. I sat up thinking about all the wonderful things I had done in the past few years, and I knew there was still so much that I wanted to do. About 40 odd minutes passed and then I seemed to find some calm and I felt a sense of contentment again. I don't like dwelling on things for too long and feeling sorry for myself, but I guess sometimes you just need to sit and cry it all out and have that moment of release. It wasn't going to do me any good to keep holding all my feelings in and trying to be this brave and happy person that I projected all the time, and I knew it would only put extra stress on my body to do so. There is only so much pretence that even I can cope with before I break, and thankfully it happened in the confinement of my own home.

The next few days I was back to my happy self and doing nice things that would make me feel relaxed. I ensured I listened to plenty of chilled music, had a candlelit bath and did things such as deep breathing. These few days were extremely uncomfortable for me and although I continued to do positive things to aid my dilemma, I longed for the scan date to arrive so we could get results and the ball rolling quickly to try and get me fixed.

August 9th was to be a busy day and I took along my parents. It started that morning with my first appointment in the General Hospital's CT imaging suite. The CT chest scan was booked in for 09:10, and this set of Xray pictures were to check that the cancer had not spread to other organs between my stomach to the chest area.

Then at 10.30 I had a meeting at the Macmillan Centre within the hospital for a wig fitting. Although I was set in my mind that I would embrace the hair loss and have my head shaved once it began to fall out, I still thought it would be a good idea to go try out the wigs. Just being at the Macmillan Centre and talking to people lifts you. I made the most of this session and enjoyed the moment with the wig fitter and my parents trying various hair colours and styles. The variety of cuts and colours they offer for the wigs is wide. Cancer patients get money up to a certain value so it is not such a big blow for anyone who wanted to purchase more than one or they could get a wig up to that amount.

As the wig fitter and my parents looked on, I decided to check out the shoulder length Jenifer Aniston style haircut with kind of blonde and brown tones. What girl would not want to look like her? Then I saw a slightly shorter blonde choppy looking wig with longer layers at the bottom, cropped in and down the neck, with top layers chopped into it. Very stylish I thought. If I was going to purchase a wig, then this was the one. I knew I would not wear it but as I have a photography fancy-dress photo booth, I knew it would end up getting good use.

12.15 came and I was back sitting with mum and dad in the oncology waiting area to have a follow up appointment with Dr Green. This was to have a chat about my chemotherapy and the chest scans. I had braced myself for this meeting, yet the news was good, the chest scans showed as being clear. That was one less thing to worry about. We discussed the type of chemotherapy that would be tailored specifically to me and when we would think about starting this.

From what I have learned, there are around two-hundred types of cancers for which there are many cocktails of cancer treatments made up and tailored to every individual's needs. We are all built differently, and our bodies have different blood types, genes, immune systems, bones, skin, hair; we also feel differently and react differently. What might work for one person may not work for another. For example, if someone was diagnosed with the same cancer as me, it doesn't necessarily mean they will be given the same chemotherapy drugs as me due to their body make-up, age, and their state of health at the time.

I do feel it is important to share knowledge to give others an insight into the unknown, which is what it feels like when you are first told such news. Learning from another's experience can help you to ask questions about your diagnosis to your own medical team about how they can help you to treat and hopefully rid you of this disease, all the time remembering that one person's treatment is tailored to that individual.

Today there are many more drugs that have been researched and trialled that are good cancer maintenance drugs to help shrink and keep cancers under control or can stop the cancer completely. I understand that some people will go through treatment after treatment and operation after operation to the extent they can no longer physically or mentally take any more. They get to the point where they have had enough and feel the need to stop. I feared what would be for me, and I felt that if drugs and operations were offered to me that would help me to continue to live a longer and healthier life, then I'd be all in!

Chemotherapy treatment is tailored specifically to that person's needs alone, and each person's cocktail of chemo drugs will be made up on the day upon the patient's arrival to the oncology ward.

Why not prep this all before, I hear you ask?

I noticed that the hospital staff put in a lot of time and effort to get people booked in on certain dates for their chemotherapy treatments. This includes doing pre-treatment bloods and weight a couple of days beforehand, to check if the patient's white blood cells are up enough to have the treatment that week. If not, this means their immune system is too low to recover from one treatment to the next, and the staff will need to discuss what is best for that patient and if the treatment should go ahead or be re-booked in later, once the white cells have had more time to rise. Prepping this way, and not making up the chemotherapy treatments in advance gives the medical staff time to assess their patient and re-arrange a different treatment date and book another ward chair for the patient.

Different patients have different time durations for treatment. Some will attend for an hour and for some it could be five hours. Some will be monthly; some will have to go for chemotherapy weekly or daily. I feel there is a lot involved in getting this done correctly and in a timely manner to ensure the treatment process runs smoothly for the patient and the team on the day. It might mean a little waiting around for the staff to get your cocktail ready but, and I see that leaving this right up to the day to be sure the patient is well enough to attend, it really works and is in the patient's best interests.

My time at the hospital was becoming more and more regular and during one of my clinics with Dr Green, a lady called Jo Wood was introduced to me. She talked to me regarding considering having some BRCA testing.

BRCA1 and BRCA2 testing is a blood test that does NOT test for cancer itself but checks for changes (mutations) in your genes. In most people cancer occurs by chance, and in a minority of people with ovarian or breast cancer, cancer occurs because they carry a genetic alteration in the BRCA1 or BRCA2 gene. These genetic alterations result in an increased lifetime risk of developing breast and ovarian cancer in women and prostate or possible breast cancer in men.

By a person having these tests and knowing whether a person carries an alteration in BRCA1 and BRCA2, it gives the cancer team more information about that person's cancer. The test results can help the doctors to make decisions and recommendations about the kind of treatments or surgery that would be most suitable to that person. The test results also give the doctors information about a person's risk of developing cancer in the future.

When asked if I would consider taking part in these tests, it was a no brainer for me, and I agreed to have them done. My biggest reason being my family, because if the results came back as having a harmful mutation, then it would be a green light for me to inform my family members to go and be tested. I chose to be a "guinea pig" for two reasons: to benefit me and my family in any way possible and to make a difference to other people's lives.

The tests came under a research study which would help to benefit others in the future. This was called Forcee and BRCA Protect Study. These small tests did not hurt or harm in any way and consisted of taking my bloods, a cervical smear, and mouth swabs. I saw this as a tiny price to pay to help to give something back to medical research.

The first step was to get the paperwork completed with Jo, after my clinic time with Dr Green.

"Okay Jackie if you would like to come with me now," Jo gestured for me to follow her with my parents in tow. We said our goodbyes to Dr Green and off we went.

My parents sat back in the waiting area and then Jo and another nurse accompanied me to a small room further down just off the waiting area and shut the door behind us. My parents sat patiently in the solemn waiting area for a few moments whilst I was completing the authorisation forms when they heard a loud roar of laughter bellowing out from the room, like a group of cackling kookaburras.

The atmosphere lightened in the waiting area and a couple of people smirked. Mum turned to dad quietly and said, "I bet that girl has gone and told them about the enema incident with the male nurse", and they both laughed. Yep! Mum got that one right and I sure had told those nurses that embarrassing story! I won't be living that one down for a long time to come but at least it gave the nurses something to laugh about and put smiles on the faces of people sitting in the waiting area.

My test results came back negative which was good. This meant it was not hereditary and there was not a chance my immediate family could have this.

Although I think of America as my second home with my second family, since my journey began, the hospital has now very much become my second home, and my illness a fact of life for me. I did not mind that I must keep having monthly check ups and clinics if it meant the hospital and drugs could help me stay alive and kicking for as long as I can.

Chapter Five

Macmillan

I was attending the Macmillan Centre workshop, Look Good Feel Better. This workshop is aimed at women to entice them to come and try a make-up session. Even if you know how to put make up on it is worth a visit just to meet others in your situation and feel a bit pampered for the day.

This is something I was glad I had chosen to do, and if I got there and didn't like it, then I still had the choice to leave if I wanted to.

Although I had accepted the fact that I was going to be losing my long curly hair once chemotherapy started, I wanted to go along and join in with other cancer sufferers to try something different and maybe enjoy the afternoon and share ideas. I thought I might learn something new I could add to my make-up regime to make me feel that little bit more feminine once my hair loss started. I wanted to attend something that would give me a boost, where I could meet others in a similar situation and maybe learn something from it.

I arrived in plenty of time and took a seat at the table to wait for more women to arrive. At each place setting on the table sat a pretty make-up bag ready for every person taking part. Eventually the other women attending began to arrive, one by one. Five of us had turned up ready to start our transformation for the afternoon. We sat around a rectangular shaped table, waiting for others to arrive.

To my right was a woman wearing a beautiful multi-coloured dupatta style head scarf. She was noticeably quiet, and when she did speak, she was very softly spoken. She stressed to the beauticians that she wanted to come along to see what Look Good Feel Better was about and how to apply make-up, but she didn't want to try out the products during the session and asked if she could take her bag of goodies away with her to try in the comfort of her own home.

Opposite us were two other women, probably mid to late fifties. At the foot of the table to my left was a girl who I seemed to hit it off with straight away, who, like myself, had suffered a previous loss in her family through cancer - it had taken her mother. While we were waiting for a couple more people to show, and the other three ladies were making conversation between themselves this girl asked me about how my journey had started and what I was feeling. I explained how it started and that I had decided to just go with it and stay positive and hopeful. I spoke of wanting to enjoy what time I might have and get through all this with my family and close friends as best as we could. We chatted for a bit and asked each other a lot of questions about our circumstances. This girl had been clear for a few years but secondary breast cancer had recently returned. We talked about her mother, who also endured the same illness and was unfortunately unable to fight it. As the girl spoke to me, she could not contain herself and began to cry.

At that moment we paused, looked at each other and something inside me caved and I could not hold in my emotions. I felt my lip start to quiver as I tried hard not to get upset but I began to cry with her, and we both reached out, put our arms around each other and hugged. We then held hands for a bit and just looked at each other. Although this was a moment of sadness between us, that hug also gave us some comfort. I didn't know this girl and yet this awful disease had brought us together sharing a very emotional moment.

Just then, there was a knock at the door and it was thrust open. We both sat back, wiped the tears from our faces and smiled at each other.

Then, out of the blue she looked at me and said, "you are just amazing; your attitude towards this is what is going to help you get through it; you seem very strong".

I smiled back with raised eyebrows as if to say "really?" but I never said anything; I couldn't, or I would have been a complete mess again.

To this day I don't know how her journey continued and if she is still living her next chapter. All I know is that having that moment with her made me realise just how serious it was and how frightened I was of the unknown. I really was scared, but I was also very focused on facing cancer head on.

I looked over my right shoulder to see another girl breezing through the door to join us. She was very petite, with gorgeous healthy glowing skin and a beautiful vibrant face. She wore a floaty, silk dress that reached to the knee, and was razorback at the top, tied at the back with the silk hanging down the back of her dress. She also wore a head scarf, which was tied like a bandana, with the long bits left hanging down the back of her neck. I thought she looked very stylish with a kind of chic/boho look about her. I sat there watching her, thinking *how can someone living with cancer and going through treatment with total loss of hair, look this good? ...* and this was before the make-up regime we were about to embark on! I thought some more - *hmmm, maybe I could go for that sort of a look when my hair falls out?*

As I looked around the room at these amazing women of different ages and personalities I was in awe, listening to their various stories, some with secondary cancer like the girl whose mother had passed and was now battling this nightmare herself for the second time, and those of us who were new to all this. I realised that although we were all feeling quite vulnerable, we weren't ready to let cancer take our lives; we were standing up to cancer by getting up and getting out and trying something to give us a purpose.

"Okay ladies let's get started" said one of the beauticians who was chairing the session. "We have one more joining us. She's currently having her treatment here but she'll join us when she can."

The beautician asked us all to open the make-up bags in front of us. We each had a variety of products to use, and I could see they were really good quality items. We were guided step by step through a cleansing regime and how to apply make-up and colours to suit our individual skin tones.

We had fun putting on the make-up and commenting on each other as we went along. The Macmillan Centre is one of those places where it doesn't matter who you are, where you come from, if you know how to apply make-up or not, if you laugh or have tears, because you are all there for the same reason and you all understand each other.

There was another knock on the door and in came a nurse wheeling in a younger girl in a wheelchair. This was the girl who had just had her treatment. Her head was bowed down looking into her lap and a blanket was tucked in around her from her waist down. She said nothing and didn't feel well enough to want to be involved. She looked so pale and fragile. We all kept the conversation light-hearted and continued to try the various cosmetics to change our appearance. All the time we were doing this, I was conscious of the young, frail, pale looking girl, who seemed to be so distant from the rest of us and was probably feeling so sick from her treatment that she felt unable to join in. It hurt me to the core to see her this way and it made me think about what might be in store for me. I knew deep down that I was not going to give in easily to cancer, and I hoped that I could fight this no matter how tough it might get.

As I was chatting and putting different colours on my face, I kept looking around at the strong, beautiful women sat in the room with me who each came along to try on the make-up, even if we weren't all in the right head space to want a bit of fun. We were all on our own personal journeys, all of which could have totally different outcomes, and I would probably never see any of these people again in my life.

There would be people like this young girl who felt too sick to join in, or the lady in the dupatta style head scarf who didn't want to use the make-up whilst sat amongst a group of strangers. People going through this may not have the energy to participate or might also feel scared of showing their emotions or talk to a bunch of people they've only just met even if they are going through the same experience as them. Some people may have feelings about the loss of hair and feel ugly or ashamed of the way they look. Maybe they fear what is to come for them or how the treatment might make them look or feel further down the line, and feel 'what is the point in trying'?

For me, doing things like this was proving I was willing to try. It was about not giving in to cancer and not giving up my life before I'd even tried. It was about finding the courage to go out of my comfort zone, to get up, get out, and try something different with people in a similar situation. I felt it was about trying to make the most of what I had, yet ensuring I did the right things such as resting, not exerting myself too much and eating the right foods. I knew all these things would help me on my road to recovery, to getting well again. I might be living with cancer but, that didn't mean I couldn't live my life. I had to keep a good balance, allow myself the odd treat occasionally and keep focused on the end goal.

The cool boho chick looked like she was embracing it and she greatly amused the group with her stories and made me giggle. She told the group about the different wigs she had purchased to wear. Some long, some short and various colours. This girl was fully making the most of her hair loss and said that her husband felt like he was sleeping with a different woman every night. She certainly was standing up to cancer in a big way and I really admired her spirit.

The Macmillan Centre is a good neutral place to go if you don't know who to talk to, or just want some you time away from the everyday stuff. It's a very welcoming and relaxed atmosphere, and this is where I found the information for the Look Good Feel Better workshop. They are there to support anyone affected by cancer: you, your family, your friends. Even if you just want to go there for a cuppa and a chat, it is somewhere you can go to talk to others and share experiences. No one judges you there and I have always been made to feel very welcome.

This centre also offers a set of free therapeutic treatments for cancer sufferers and of course the wig service. I noticed they have a room there called The Bluebell Room. This had an array of head scarfs and hats for men, women, and children to try and see what might be suitable for them.

The staff at the Macmillan Centre are supportive and offer treatments, counselling, and advice on things like employment benefits. They will also advise on such things as writing to your energy suppliers to help with your circumstances, such as temporarily decreasing bill payments, changing tariffs, or sending out such things to help you manage when you start to become weak from treatment – things you wouldn't normally think could be available to you, like rubber lid openers.

My nearest Macmillan Centre is situated at the Southampton General Hospital. I recommend anyone affected by cancer or who is with someone receiving cancer treatment, should at least find their nearest cancer centre and go check it out. Most provide therapy treatments, leaflets with information and books on how to eat well and lead as normal life as you can.

The thing is, no one ever financially saves for something as serious as cancer. You never expect to encounter anything like this, so it is not the sort of thing you have a money pot for. Cancer can hit you hard financially, especially if you need a great deal of time off work. Macmillan and other organisations can give you advice on all this, even if you feel you don't need it, it's worth paying them a visit just to talk it through with someone. They might discuss things that you may not have thought about where your finances are concerned, such as how to get a grant to help cushion reduced wages or where to seek advice to get help with paying your bills.

There are many good places all over the country that are there to help you, so my advice is seek them out and use them! When you are at hospital ASK! They will be able to point you in the right direction. Google cancer charities and use the information at the back of my book as a place to start if you need to.

Some charities may ask for a small money donation or will have a little donation box within their practice. People are not obliged to donate; however, they are there in case you feel like you want to give something back and you don't have to break the bank to do it. Every penny counts and even just the smallest donation means so much to these wonderful people who donate their time, patience, and kindness to be there for those of us who need it most.

I occasionally make money donations when I can afford to or I like to take along to my visit's things like a box of tea bags, a packet of biscuits or jar of coffee to leave there for them. This all helps these charities in some way to provide that little something extra in their service to visitors to their centres who go there for help. I think a good cuppa and talking my worries through with someone outside my close network makes it all seem a bit easier and I can get it clearer in my own head. It is a release for me and on occasion I let the tears flow, which stops me holding it all inside.

Another way to donate is by doing a service for the charity. I love my photography and even before I was diagnosed with cancer, I would go along to the Great South Run every year to photograph it for free for Macmillan. I still do in between my treatments.

Penny Brohn is another cancer charity situated in Bristol which my friend Tess told me about. Tess is a friend who has been through the mill and back with many cancer treatments and operations. She has been zapped and cut from here to Timbuktu and she is still living a happy and fruitful life.

I met Tess through my friend, Jo. She is Jo's sister and she instantly inspired me with her story. Tess is a fun, gutsy, brave, and inspirational character, who has such a zest for life that she was not going to let cancer rule it in any way, shape, or form. When I first got cancer, I thought about what Tess had endured and I sure as hell was going to try to do the same. At that time Tess was still coming through it all in her recovery and back and forth for hospital check-ups.

Tess told me of a retreat she did at Penny Brohn for a couple of days with Jo back in July of 2015, whilst she was going through her cancer ordeal. She said that Penny Brohn was one of the best things she had done and recommended I should go there myself. I will talk more about Tess later in this story because she really inspired me to be the stronger person I am today.

From June right up until my chemotherapy treatment I suffered symptoms such as shortness of breath, some chest pains, bloated stomach, struggling with constipation and experiencing just a watery fluid and various discharges from my body. This was all due to the tumours pushing on my organs and the fluid build-up in my stomach. My poor body took a lot of weight and stress and did not know at times if it was coming or going.

I just wanted to get the ball rolling and get something sorted. It's not nice waiting for test results and treatment to commence. It's probably the worst part because it's time spent thinking, worrying, and feeling uncomfortable, and probably the stress wasn't helping my situation. It wasn't nice for my family either. I kind of felt like it was wasted time and I wanted to start my treatment sooner rather than later. I understand that there are many people like me waiting to be seen and the hospital have a duty of care to all their patients and need to ensure all the necessary tests are done correctly leading up to the patient's treatment. However, it was the agonising wait and the questions in my mind of *what if the cancer is still growing at a fast rate during this time? Or what if the tumours cause my insides to erupt/burst and sepsis sets in and poisons me?*. I guess I was thinking way outside the box there but thinking about such possibilities can really make your mind work overtime.

The next day I had my bloods and weight taken prior to my chemotherapy treatment. Normally a CA125 red blood count is under thirty-five however, mine was at eight hundred and sixty point forty which was far from being a good sign. After all, I did have advanced Stage 3 ovarian cancer. There was no way I was allowing the test results to scare me into submission. I feared the worst, but I didn't want my mind to go on a downward spiral. I chose to keep focused on the now and dealt with it each day.

Nobody knows what cards they are going to be dealt in life, and most of us don't know at the time we are told such news of how little or long we could have left. Some of us are good at reading our own bodies and being able to tell if what we are feeling is not right, but I honestly believe in not giving up hope and to try treatments to see how we respond.

We won't all react the same way or have the same outcome and I am fearful that these cancer cells could become wise to the maintenance drugs, and we will have to try something else to supress the cancer if this happens. I do believe I need to keep positive, not stress too much over the future as to what might or might not be, and just get on with living my life. So as long as my body responds well to the maintenance treatments that are offered to me, then I will keep experimenting with them to keep myself alive and kicking.

Chapter Six

Intravenous

Drugs Day is nigh! Fiona arrived at my flat on the Thursday evening after work. She brought me some jasmine tea and a homemade cottage pie, courtesy of her partner, Andy, so that once Fi arrived at my home, we could both chill out for the evening without the hassle of cooking.

After our dinner, Fi and I relaxed for a few hours and then settled down for the night. The morning ahead was to be my very first chemotherapy cycle, and I didn't know what to expect at the hospital. Although I was feeling calm, I lay there in my bed anticipating what it was all going to be like and how it might make me feel. It took a while for sleep to come but when it did, I slept right through.

Friday August 12th, 2016, C Level Oncology, Bay C, Chair 4, and D Day had arrived! The alarm went off at 6.30am and I got up and made us coffee whilst Fi took a shower. Once we were both dressed and ready to go, we checked off everything I had in my chemo bag. It was no surprise to Fi that I had packed all bar the kitchen sink. To be fair, I have always been known as a bit of a "bag lady" and probably didn't need half of what I had packed however, I had spent hours online researching the kinds of things cancer patients take with them or might need during treatment.

See reference pages at the back of the book

Once parked, we made our way into the hospital, Fi carrying my two large bags whilst I walked in like a little diva with my 'entourage'. Fi joked about the bags I had.

"Hey," I said, "I need one alone for food," and I looked at her with a cheeky grin.

"No surprise there then; what the bloody hell is in the other one?" she laughed.

"My comfy gear and entertainment. Well, I am a chemo virgin, so I would rather rock up with too much stuff than not enough."

We walked from the car park into the building and up to oncology on C Level. Me, myself, and my entourage (AKA Fiona) arrived at the main oncology reception. I introduced myself and said I'd arrived to check in for my first chemotherapy session in the day unit. The receptionist looked up and smiled and asked us to walk to our left and through another set of doors. We did so, then buzzed the intercom and waited. I was feeling okay but slightly anxious. I felt like Fi could read me.

She brushed my arm, "you okay honey?" I smiled and nodded.

"Can I help you?" came a voice from the intercom. "Yes, my name is Jacqueline Ridout, I am here for my treatment today."

"Okay Jacqueline, come on through." The door clicked for us to enter the treatment area.

The door is a secure buzz entry to ensure the hospital can manage the amount of traffic in and out of the treatment area, thus keeping the area safely contained and prevents cancer patients who may have a low white blood count (immune system) from possibly catching anything. The hospital only allows one person in with you when having treatment to keep the treatment area numbers to a minimum and ensures the comfort and modesty of each cancer patient

The nurses showed Fiona and me to my chair in the room. Mine was a leather looking recliner chair and Fi had a chair nearby to sit with me. I had a side cabinet to put some of my things and thankfully room to put my large bags packed with my home comforts and lots of nice food to eat throughout. I had googled on the internet prior to my chemotherapy treatment to see what sort of things would be good to pack for such feelings as nausea, etc. I wanted things I liked and a mixture of sweet and bland foods, just in case I felt I needed it to help with the sickness feeling from the drugs. Better to have too much than to worry about having too little. I also took my own bottle of water as I didn't want to be feeling dehydrated, although they did have water on tap for us to use.

We sat waiting patiently whilst the nurses retrieved and checked off the first lot of drugs to be prescribed to me. Fiona asked what I might want from my cool bag, and we took out a couple of things to put on the cabinet to the side of my chair. I also took out a neck pillow, fluffy bed socks and blanket should I need them.

Throughout my chemotherapy we watched as the nurses worked non-stop throughout the day, going from one person to the next. Occasionally you hear of people who moan about the NHS but, I have to say, I really do have to take my hat off to the oncology team. The nurses, doctors, administration staff and surgeons all work tirelessly to help people. There are also those working in the background at the hospital such as those working in the hospital shops, porters, ambulance teams, cleaners, people filling the vending machines - they all play a part in the hospital process. I truly could not do what these amazing people do day in and day out. They attend to people who may not know if they will get through this, they see how sick they each become with the treatment, yet through the stress of it all I don't know how they can refrain from showing their feelings. These medical people deal with a variety of personalities each experiencing a range of emotions. These emotions and feelings can usually start with shock, fear, sadness, anger, frustration, disbelief, rejection, a sense of giving up or a sense of wanting to fight. For some, emotions will change throughout treatment and cancer can sometimes change you as a person and your outlook on life moving forwards. I don't think there is a wrong or right way that anyone should feel or how to deal with it.

With the medical teams, they must treat everyone on a par, so to speak, by not showing too much emotion when they must tell someone they have an illness or worse. I think it is by far one of the hardest and most demanding jobs in the world to do. Many people lean on the medical teams for support and just attending one of my sessions or a clinic, made me realise just how many people are suffering and living with cancer. The turnover of people in and out of the oncology area for blood tests, chemo, to discuss their outcomes with their consultant, etc seems endless and I saw the medical team dealing with what must have been hundreds of people a day, all with different cancers, all with different treatments and all with quite different outcomes.

Every time a new pill was given to me or a new chemo bag was put on my canula, the nurses would repeatedly ask me the same questions: name, DOB and first line of my address. It was second nature to them and probably vital they do this to ensure every time they were giving the correct cocktail to the correct patient and a good way of checking our response to make sure we were doing okay whilst in their care.

I was there for day treatment, and some were there for a couple of hours. There were also some people with asbestos related cancers who took a daily visit to the hospital for their short hour treatments. The traffic of cancer patients going through that ward really opened my eyes up as to just how many are affected and this was just adults. The children's ward was separate.

Firstly, anti-sickness pills were given. I was told to also use these to take just for a couple days after treatment and occasionally thereafter as I needed them. Taking them regularly can cause constipation, which I felt I had endured enough leading up to my treatment!

The first drip to go in the canula inserted to the back of my hand was the saline – this was to flush the vein through my body for approximately fifteen minutes. This keeps you hydrated and helps the chemo drugs get to the right place in your body. A Piriton anti-allergy was injected via another tube to prevent any allergic reactions to the chemo drugs, such as a rash, itching, shortness of breath, swelling to face, dizziness, etc.

Once hooked up and the saline process was under way, we sat back and let it take its course. I started to feel a bit strange. I had a cold feeling from the saline slowly working into my veins. I could feel the coolness creeping through.

My first of the two chemo solutions I had was called Paclitaxel. Paclitaxel is mainly used to treat such cancers as ovarian, breast and non-small cell lung cancer.

The nurse came by with her tray and started to prep me for this next stage with the Paclitaxel drug.

"Jacqueline this will be drip fed over the next 3 hours. If you experience any stinging or burning sensations that become too uncomfortable then please let us know as soon as possible.".

All wired up and ready to go. Fi and I sat chatting and chilling and she would occasionally ask if I needed anything from my numerous bags. Slowly I began to feel a warm sensation, which seemed to stay with me for some time. There was a gradual rise in my temperature and then a feeling of coldness with it, a bit like that white-out feeling you get when you're drunk or experiencing a feeling of passing out. I guess I might have been feeling a bit of nausea and my body was probably reacting to this first-time of receiving the drugs.

"Jac, are you okay honey?"

"Yes Fi, just feel rather hot and cold all at once and a bit sick, but I'm sure it will pass." Fi went to fill up my water bottle. As I watched her, I thought about everything she does, not just for me but our group of friends. Fi likes to take charge most of the time. If we go away for a weekend, she is on the case researching where to go and what to do, and she is literally all over it with organising things. We have all shared many good memories together over the years.

Cancer is very intrusive and uninvited but I welcomed the chemo in the hope it would help me to rid my body of the cancer so I could then concentrate afterwards on building my resilience back up and feel well again. Having her support took my mind off things a bit and made the time go quickly.

After this another saline flush was given to me to flush back through my system for approximately 5 to 10 minutes. During my time there, I had got up a few times to use the toilet, as I was drinking a lot of fluids to keep well hydrated and to help with the sicky feelings that came and went.

To do this, each patient must unplug their machine, and wheel the attached drugs to the toilet with them. As I stood up from my chair, I realised my trousers felt stuck to my skin and I noticed that my seat was wet, yet I had felt nothing during the saline flush or the treatment going through my body. Fi and I, thinking it was pee, could not smell anything and when I wiped the seat the fluid was not discoloured in any way. I couldn't understand this and put it down to my muscles having been so relaxed and probably a numbness in my body, that I felt absolutely nothing.

I called the nurse to query this and to explain that I didn't feel like I was peeing, and she told me that this sometimes happens, and the saline will flush straight through me; because of this I decided I needed to do a list of what things to think about bringing to a chemotherapy session to help others , such as large sanitary pads, to ensure the comfort of the patient during treatment and any little accidents like this. You see again, because everyone reacts differently, we might not all experience the same things; however, I believe in sharing knowledge of what happened to me to prep anyone going for their first chemotherapy treatment. I guess the nurses and doctors never thought to highlight this, and maybe because it is something that no one really wants to talk about due to embarrassment.

Then on to the second chemo drip infusion of Carboplatin for an hour. This was kept covered in a red bag to stop light contamination. Carboplatin is the most used drug to treat ovarian cancer and is the most effective.

The drugs did give me a kind of high feeling, which I was not expecting, or going to complain about, as I needed to feel as relaxed as possible after the anticipation of the day. I noticed my temperature dropping and then rising slightly and I kept putting my blanket around me then taking it back off again. I kept sweeping in and out of a kind of sickness feeling, and I could feel a tingling sensation through the tips of my fingers. Then I had a sense of drowsiness. I had all this happening to me which gave me the kind of feeling you have when you have had too much alcohol, a kind of white out/vertigo feeling.

I had a slight cooling sensation as the drugs were being fed into my body and a strange taste in my mouth, a bit like a metallic taste.

The nurse advised Fiona she could walk down to the Pharmacy to collect my drugs prescription for me whilst I was dosed up with my cocktail of chemo. This would be to take home and follow.

"I know this sounds ignorant of me," I said interrupting the nurse mid-sentence, "but do you think you can find out what my blood type is for me please as I don't know this".

The nurse turned to me and said, "yes of course. It won't be done today as it is nearing the end of your session and I have other patients that I need to attend to, but we can find this out for you next time you come to the clinic, or your next chemotherapy session". She then went on to explain that most patients are not sick on the chemotherapy and will feel tiredness and mainly groggy afterwards. It's a well-tolerated treatment. The drugs are less toxic and not the nasty ones. She said that these days the medicines are much better and have come a long way from what they once were.

There will always be the chemo horror stories floating around and I see that a lot of people never hear the good things. It's the same for many things in life, such as when a woman gives birth; they always want to tell their horror stories of all the things that didn't go right or the amount of pain they were in. I guess those people who do okay and do cope are the ones whose stories you seldom hear about. The majority of women I know have coped well. I think when people go through such painful or traumatic experiences that these are the things they tend to remember more because we are more affected by them.

I had a few hiccups along the way too, but you know what? I don't think the minor things such as a student nurse pricking my skin about eight or nine times warrants a complaint when the NHS are doing all that they can to save me and prolong my life. We all make mistakes in life whether it be in our personal lives or our professional work. No one is perfect and sometimes people must take a step back and look at the bigger picture and put things into a bit more perspective.

Another saline flush was then given to me, and finally taking out the cannula from my hand and school was out.

The actual treatment was not as bad as I thought it was going to be and lasted around 5/6 hours including getting me set up. Once Fi had my aftercare drugs and the nurse got round to unhooking me and giving me aftercare advice along with a twenty-four-hour hotline number, we were free to leave. The phone number was in case I experienced any reactions post treatment, or that my temperature should rise above thirty-seven point five.

I noticed post chemo treatment I had a feeling of achy bones, I was very lethargic, suffered occasional headaches and achiness to the kidney area so I would up my water intake to ensure I kept well hydrated. For a couple of days my face would feel warm and sensitive, and I would have a slight itching to my skin.

Two days went by and by the Sunday I had become slightly groggy and feeling a bit rough around the edges. My struggle with still trying to go to the toilet varied. This was only after one chemo cycle, so I guess I could not hold out for miracles just yet. I looked at my stomach and it seemed bigger, and my legs were still painful. This was not going to be an overnight fix and maybe my worries and expectations were running a little high. This was going to take time for the chemo to do its work and shrink my tumours down.

Today was the day I was going to get myself out for a bit of exercise and pay a visit to Monkey World, an ape rescue centre to meet one of the park workers, Shelley. She had viewed some of my photography work and we had arranged via email for me to go there to meet her and donate a canvas to Monkey World for auctioning at one of their charity events.

Shelley, like me, has experienced cancer in her life. Shelley spoke of her mother, who was at that time, going through it and was not doing too great. It was a sunny day and my drive down to Monkey World was an easy straight forward one. I arrived at the entrance turnstiles and was greeted by Shelley. Before I ventured into the park, we sat at their onsite café and talked for quite some time about how this was affecting Shelley's family, and I learned and understood so much about what Shelley and her family were all going through. Having an illness is a massive blow on a person's life. It prevents your ability to do things, it takes your working life from you, it weighs down on those in your life who are going through this horrid journey with you, and it crushes the hearts of those who have lost loved ones. I could see how much it meant to Shelley to want her mother to get well and yet, even though she was holding on to hope, she seemed at a loss as to what was going to happen next.

I explained to Shelley about my love for Monkey World and it being a haven for me. A place where I can stroll round, take pictures if I wish and just watch these beautiful creatures and their different personalities coming through. When there, I like to take my time at the various enclosures and sometimes I feel as if I am engaging in a way with some of the primates. Some will copy your repetitive actions and are very playful and some just sit there staring, as if looking right into your eyes and deep into your soul; because of what this amazing place does and how it makes me feel, I try to show the primates' emotions within my photography, and I think I have achieved this in some of the work I have produced through my time at Monkey World.

Listening to Shelley's story touched me and really opened me up to what her family was going through at that time. Upon leaving the park I prayed in my heart and I wished in my mind for her mother to be well again. Before starting up the engine, I sat in my car for a few minutes just thinking about what a rubbish time cancer gives to people.

The trip to Monkey World wiped me out and when Monday came and I was in bed with my legs elevated and hot water bottles on my stomach due to the uncomfortable feeling again. Due to being awake during the night and feeling terrible, I decided to call the medical twenty-four-hour phone line. They told me to take Senna laxative and to call the Macmillan nurses in the morning to talk further should I need them. The laxative didn't do much to alleviate the discomfort I felt and I knew I had to try and ride this out. Another couple of days and I was in for my wig fitting at the hospital. Again, this was back at the wonderful Macmillan Centre. I knew from day one, when I was told I would lose my hair, that I would for sure NOT be wearing a wig. I guess everyone to their own, and for me, I just wanted to go with it and embrace whatever came my way on my journey.

I have spoken of how hair loss, especially for women, is such a big deal. Women like to feel good about themselves and look good. The thing with the hair loss is that once this happens, it happens all over your body and face, and then you get near to the end of your treatment and you can start to look sick, so all this combined, can understandably make a woman feel very unattractive and lose confidence.

Through my time at hospital and having talked to other women about how they were trying to come to terms with hair loss, it also made me feel that there are just as many men and children who also go through illness and body changes and might also go through similar experiences or have these feelings. Anyone experiencing cancer in their life, even if they are at the hospital to support a person with cancer, should go and visit their local Cancer Centre; just do it. I found the Macmillan Centre in Southampton not only do the Look Good Feel Better programme, and the wig fitting appointments, they also give advice and have examples of various head wear, which you can purchase from different companies and on the internet. They give free holistic treatments to those who need it such as reflexology, aromatherapy massage, Indian head massage, Reiki, and give counselling to both the patient and their loved ones. You are under no obligation to go, but I feel it is worth popping your head round the door and you will be greeted by the friendly face of someone you can talk to.

This whole thing can be quite daunting at first when you experience changes, let alone go out of your comfort zone to go to a place that you didn't choose to be at. But here is a place of calm and a place where you can just go for some quiet time or to sit and offload all your worries to someone if you feel the need. They do not pressure you into anything you do not feel you want to do or speak about. The people who work here will understand, as many of them will have experienced cancer themselves. They are best placed to give advice and just be there for you to talk, chill out, cry, or to arrange for a treatment to make you feel somewhat normal and good about yourself.

I believe in trying anything that will help you in some way to get through this a bit easier and release everything that is building up inside that most people cannot let go of in front of their loved ones. The Macmillan team can advise you on what would be the best therapy for you, your body, and your mind at that time.

In my case they could assess me and my needs, for instance due to the nature of my cancer and where it was, I was advised to not have massage in that area. Then I had the choice to go with just a back, neck, and shoulders massage suitable for pregnant women. This was so as not to aggravate the area in which my cancer was living, yet I could still have some of the benefits of the massage. I was sat upright on a chair and the therapist only worked on me from the back, up the neck and right to under my cranium. This took the pressure off my stomach whilst not interfering with that area in any way, shape, or form.

If you choose to go with a wig option, then the centre arranges for you to be given an amount to put towards the purchase of your wig. This way it entices people, men, children, and women, to make an appointment to at least go and try some on. It is all done discreetly in one of the adjoining rooms and they book a wig fitter to come along with various wigs and toupees for people to try to see what feels good on them and which suits best. They have been known to have people attend, who want to try something completely different or outrageous compared to what they normally have. Some have totally gone the opposite colour or hairstyle to their original one. The wig fitters can also cut and style a wig into shape for you if you feel it is a bit too long, but you like the fit, or you want it to look more layered, etc.

My treatment appointments continued every three weeks and afterwards I could feel my ovary area starting to twinge so I knew the chemo must be doing its magic. I ended up having four chemotherapy treatments in total before my full hysterectomy operation.

I endured many headaches towards the end of August, and maybe it was because I was feeding my body with less fuel due to the worry about making it worse. Due to how I was feeling, my friends Kerry and Darren asked me to go stay with them for a few days so I could relax, and they could look after me and give my parents a break.

* * *

Chapter Seven

Toupee or Not Toupee

I noticed my hair was becoming very dry and coarse and I could feel it moulting in areas. It was slowly starting to fall out in small clumps. I had not wanted to wash it because every time I tried to do anything with it, I could feel strands of it between my fingers, but it needed doing.

One morning I grabbed a towel from the cupboard and made my way to the bathroom. I undressed and got into the shower. I stood underneath the warm flowing water, cupped my hands, and began to push the warm flowing water over my face and back through my hair. I poured some shampoo into my hands and began to wash my hair, being gentle as I rubbed it into my hair and began to massage my scalp.

What was that? I thought. Then I suddenly realised I was holding a clump of my frizzy, brittle hair, entangled between my fingers. It was happening. I washed out the shampoo, leaned over to turn the water off and stepped back out on to the bathmat. As I turned around and walked towards the mirror to look at myself, I hated what I could see. It wasn't the having no hair that bothered me as I knew it was going to happen at some point, but I had clumps of hair missing in areas on my head and it looked awful. There was no way I was going to be one of those people with a comb over! It had to be all or nothing and I was not leaving it looking the way it did. I dried myself down, put my clothing back on and made my way down the stairs to find Kerry.

I pushed open the living room door.

"Kerry!"

Kerry was sitting on the sofa, she looked up, "yes honey?"

"Look! My hair is falling out in clumps, and I don't like it. I want it all shaved off."

As I held my clump of hair and continued to talk to Kerry, it was as if this whole conversation was happening in slow motion. I looked at my friend's facial expression, which was showing concentration but also concern, yet Kerry stayed calm whilst listening to me. We had a few moments together looking at the matted mess in my hands and then discussed calling her stepdaughter, Mia, who was a hairdresser, to see if she would be able to shave my head for me. Kerry made the call.

"Mia it's Kerry. Are you working today?"

Mia knew she would be getting a call from us at some point as she was fully aware of my situation and had offered to help when needed. Kerry asked Mia if she had time during that day or after work to shave the rest of my hair off. Mia obliged straight away and asked us to drive straight over to her salon.

We made our drive to the Sun Rooms, Mia's place of work, to have my head shaved. I asked Mia if she would be using clippers to do this. I felt this would be much better than using a razor as this would likely cause spotting and bleeding which I did not want in my condition. Firstly, it could cause cross-contamination and secondly, it would probably look unsightly.

"Honey, can you keep two separate locks of my curls before you brush through my hair as my parents want to keep one each?". Mia did so, and then she sat in the chair and gowned me up ready to start. Mia cut away some of the longer hair first and as she turned on the clippers to put the metal teeth to my brittle hair, I noticed Kerry looking at me. I wondered what was going through her mind and if all this was making her think back to her auntie Carol. I remember how much Kerry was affected by the loss of her auntie so this could not have been an easy task for her. It was not until that moment when Mia started shaving my head, that I realised what I had asked of Mia. It was a big deal and a really hard thing emotionally for her to have to do and I did not contemplate that although she was happy to do this favour for me that she would be also devastated by all this. I sat there in the chair, no emotion, just wanting the horrid mess removed from me. As Mia moved the clippers up my scalp, I realised that she was welling up to the point that she could not hold her feelings back and she began to cry. As Mia bent forwards, she wrapped her arms around me, and we cuddled for a moment. She could not hold back the tears and I could feel her trembling slightly.

"Jackie I can't believe this is happening to you, it's not right, this isn't fair that you have to go through all this."

We all stopped and had a moment together then a very emotional Mia managed to gather herself and she continued to work her magic on me.

I thought Kerry was being very brave about this. Kerry had been in this situation before with her auntie, and she was again going through similar, if not the same thoughts and feelings as she did a few years ago. Research has by far progressed over the last ten years compared to when Carol was with us. Various maintenance drugs are continually being tried and tested to help cancer patients to survive a bit longer or give them additional years of life.

Strangely, when the job was done, I was surprised at how much I liked it and at how good I looked bald. With the full loss of my long curly hair between my second and third chemo treatments, I realised it was not as devastating as I thought it would be for me.

Kerry commented on my head shape.

"Seriously mate, your head is perfectly round; there are no bumps or anything, just a nice round shape."

Mia began smiling and said, "you look so good with no hair, even after losing all your curls; it really suits you". Both were amused by the fact I was mincing in front of the salon mirror, enjoying my new head of nothing, looking well-polished. In fact, I looked like I could have auditioned for a part in Star Trek or something. Kerry and I could see Mia was beginning to have another emotional moment. 'My goodness', I thought, 'Mia is seriously affected by this'. We three took ourselves around to the pub next door for lunch and a glass of prosecco. Afterwards

Kerry and I said our goodbyes to Mia, and we all hugged in the car park before Mia walked back to work. It felt wrong to then leave Mia behind, probably still upset over all this rubbish.

All along it had been a scary feeling to think of losing all my long curly locks; however, this was just another part of my journey and so I chose to embrace it just like the boho chick did at the Look Good Feel Better day. I noticed that I had lost all my hair everywhere, so I guess not having to use anything such as a lady shave, blow dryer or do bikini waxing for a while was going to be less time consuming and effort.

The one thing I found strange throughout this whole process was how I dealt with this compared to how everyone around me had reacted. They were all the most supportive and loving people in the world to me, yet how devastated and upset my family and friends had been by it all. I just couldn't seem to feel upset about this and felt at some point I might have a massive meltdown, or maybe I never would. I just hoped that if I did, it would not be in a place full of people like the middle of a shopping centre. From the very beginning I was more worried about how I was first going to tell people and how my loved ones would cope receiving this news. The only time I cried was behind the curtain in the hospital when first told, because I was upset for what my parents were hearing, and about to endure. I had had a couple of moments with friends and cousins but deep down, in a strange way, I was really coping well. I think everyone is affected differently and has different coping mechanisms. This all seemed as though I was in this bubble and watching and worrying more about those who were on the outside hearing the news.

Next on my agenda was to find a look that would suit me and make me feel more feminine, so I went on a googling frenzy to find my perfect style. I wanted to try out different things and so I went on a mission ordering head scarfs. Some floral, some hippy-chick, plain ones, and some sassy, chic looking scarfs. Being a bit of a "hat girl", I also purchased a couple of soft, comfortable beanie hats and some thicker woolly beanie hats from Amazon ready for the wintertime. I wanted to ensure I had a few different types of headwear for any occasion so that I felt comfortable wherever I went. I didn't want to feel restricted because of my hair loss and I wanted many styles and colours that would suit anything in my wardrobe. I even found a beige-coloured tube-shaped piece of material which sat on the head like a beanie hat but would allow air to get to the scalp from the open part that hung at the back. This was going to be useful to wear on a spa treat my cousin Jane had planned. I needed something that didn't stand out too much and was comfortable enough to wear around the pool area without feeling hot and looking ridiculous. My friends and family also purchased and sent me many varieties of headwear to try, and I am adamant that my ever-growing stylish collection became bigger than the contents of Victoria Beckhams wardrobe!

My mood seemed to dip and I was feeling a little fed up during the week after my hair shave. I was trying to keep myself in good spirits. Probably the nausea effect of the drugs didn't help how I was feeling inside. During and after treatments the lethargy would set in, and the nausea washed slowly in and out like the tide. I guess after this I kind of knew what to expect at my future treatments. Well, I was certainly hoping I didn't feel any worse.

* * *

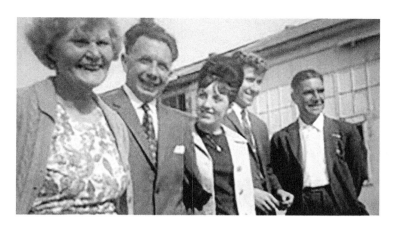

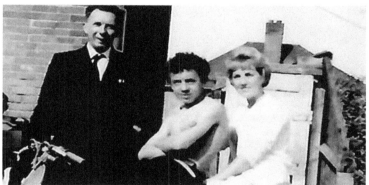

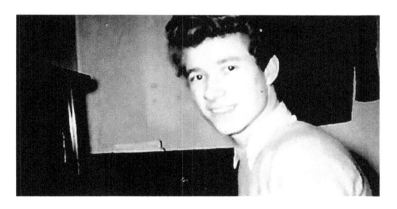

My parents with their parents.

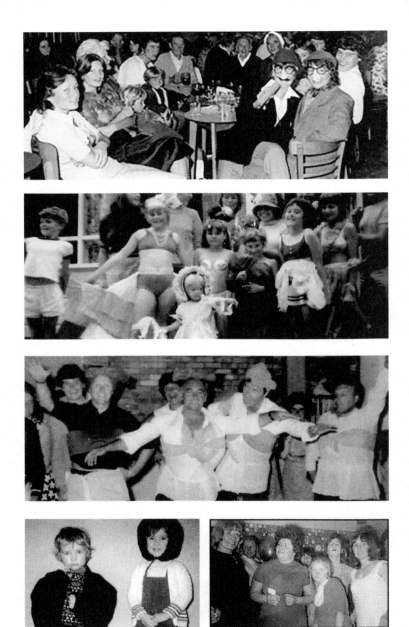

My awesome memories of my growing up and our family holidays.

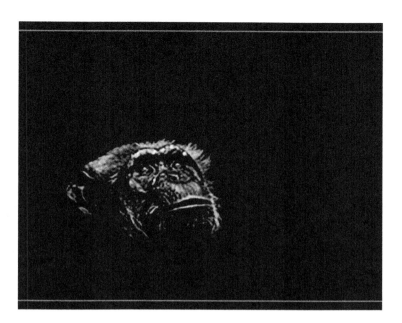

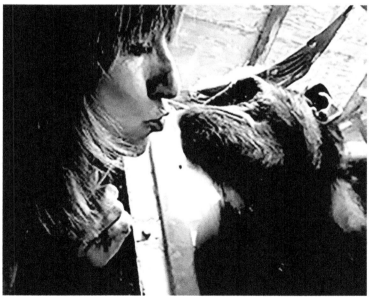

Monkey world became my haven, and my photography my soul food.

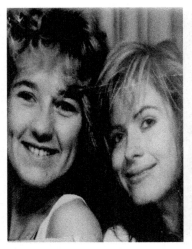
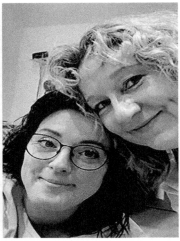
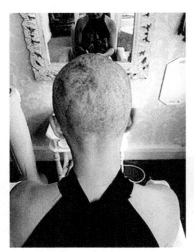
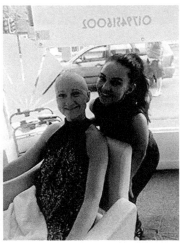

Top left: Me and Jeni my American "sister" when we were just 18
Top right: Jo, who is a beautiful person and a legend
Bottom right: Mia (Kerry's step-daughter) who shaved my hair.

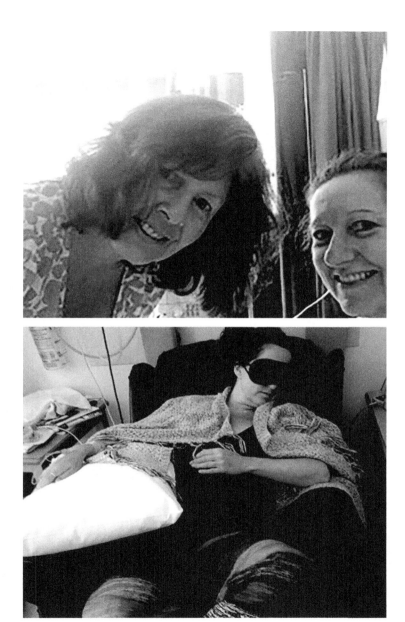

Top: *Fiona supporting me at my first chemo session.*
Bottom: *First chemo. Me asleep during treatment*

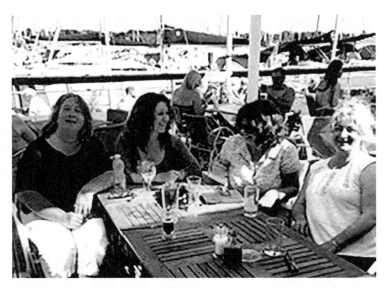

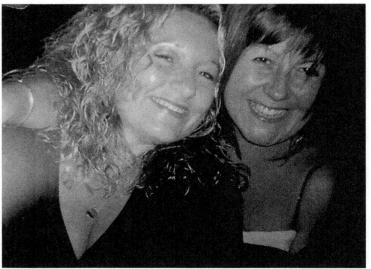

Top: Time spent with my friends at the marina. I call this shot our last supper as it was taken before I started chemo treatment.
Bottom: Mia's step-mum, Kerry, my close friend who had me to stay regular to take care of me.

Chapter Eight

B Positive

How did we get to September already? I thought time was meant to fly when you "were" having fun?! My friend, Jacquie, who had also experienced cancer first-hand, was in remission with breast cancer treatment, after having a big operation, and yet she had got in her car the night before my second chemotherapy treatment and drove down to be with me for this.

It is times like this which stick with me when I think of people in my life like Jacquie, who also have their own trauma to deal with, yet give so much love and support and will be there at the drop of a hat. I was amazed that Jacquie could put herself through this for me, knowing she was still in pain. She travelled from Birmingham all the way to Southampton, to stay overnight, and to then to sit with me the following day through my treatment, before making the long journey back home afterwards. She must have been shattered after all that, yet she arrived with a huge smile, a big warm hug and being the Miss Wonderful she always has been.

Whilst we were waiting to get set up ready for my chemo treatment, I gave Jacquie my food order and she popped to Costa in the hospital to give the nurse and I some time to get me rigged up to my machine.

Two ladies walked in, a taller lady with short dark brown hair and a shorter lady with short white hair. They sat down in the bay area to my left. The taller dark-haired lady left the room.

The nurse was getting me all set up ready for my treatment, wrapping the tourniquet nice and tight around my forearm and then slowly inserting the canula into the back of my hand before attaching the treatment drip tube to the canula. She had just turned to the side to do something when I started to feel a bit dizzy and wheezy; suddenly, I felt a rush up my body, like a hot flush with a tingly feeling. I realised I was starting to feel very faint, and my breathing became a lot faster.

I tried to gasp for air as the nurse turned around and I pointed at the tourniquet still tied around my forearm. The poor lady swung her chair around and began to undo the tourniquet. This was just a small hiccup where the tourniquet was accidentally left on for too long. Unfortunately for the nurse, my friend Jacquie walked back into the room as all this was happening and wondered what the hell was going on.

It happens, we are each human and to be honest this mishap was a lot less life threatening than what was growing inside me. Usually, it is the smallest things like this that can happen in a place like a hospital and yet some would be too quick to complain about it. But they aren't so quick in telling the NHS staff how amazing they are for doing what they do day in and day out to try to get people like me well again; hence the reason for me writing about this experience. For me it was a small hiccup and eventually I laughed it off.

The dark-haired lady had just walked back into the room and had gone to sit in the chair opposite with the lady who was there to have her treatment. Jacquie stood with toastie and coffee in hand just looking shocked.

"What's been going on here then?" she queried.

"It's okay. The nurse forgot to take the tourniquet off after canulating me."

"Oh god honey, that isn't good."

"No, it's fine, I just felt hot and thought I was going to faint, but it's okay now." Jacquie looked quite worried about it all, but as I said, it was an accident and no big deal.

As I still wanted to know what my blood type was, I queried this again with the nurse. She said she would find out and let me know.

Jacquie and I sat chatting to each other and then looked across the room to the other two ladies, who also looked back at us, and we all smiled at each other. As my treatment was just about underway, the smaller lady of the two started to cry whilst they were both waiting for her to be set up.

I really felt for her and knew she was probably feeling anxious about it all. I hate seeing people upset at the best of times, let alone in a hospital environment. Jac and I looked at each other and I felt the emotion in me, and I could also see it on Jac's face. The nurse walked over to her and proceeded to pull the curtains around where the ladies were sitting.

"No, please don't pull the curtains and segregate me from others, I'll be fine, I just need a minute," the smaller lady said.

With this the nurse left the curtains pulled back and then started to get the lady settled in ready to start her treatment. My treatment was approximately 6 hours long, whereas the treatment for the lady across from me started after mine and it was finished a lot earlier.

The nurse went over to detach her from the canula and spoke with her for a moment to ensure all was okay prior to her leaving. Both ladies started to gather their things to leave. As they did so and started to walk towards the exit door, the smaller lady walked towards me and stopped to talk.

"I love your head scarf, it really suits you. Where did you purchase it as I think I'd like to try wearing these?" she proceeded to tell me how chic it looked.

I smiled and thanked her, "I can text you the website and a few others if you like? … do you have your mobile number to hand?"

"No, I don't, my name is Gill, but this is my daughter, Sue, so can you please text the details to her?"

"I'm Jackie and of course I can."

We all chatted for a brief while and I exchanged phone numbers so I could text Sue the details. Gill had a kind and friendly face and I thought how brave she was to face her treatment head on after starting with such emotion. As soon as they left, I felt happy we had made a connection. Paths in your life, whether chosen or not can connect you to wonderful people and can bring you good friendships.

Since that day Gill, Sue and I have kept in touch, and we meet occasionally to go for walks. Through talking and getting to know Gill more, I found out she had undergone both radiotherapy and chemotherapy treatments a few years ago for breast cancer. Gill explained that the second cancer she recently had was a completely different cancer to that in the past. Gill loved to write poetry and was inspired to write a piece based on something unusual that happened during her treatments, which gave her some comfort. And so, with Gill's permission, I share this with you.

Unexpected Comfort

The operation, the stays in hospital, and the chemotherapy were over. Now the 19 visits for radiotherapy were about to begin.

I had always known that robins were cheeky, brave little birds but, the one who suddenly appeared, sat on my car, and then the following day pecked on the window, hopped into the car and stared at me, seemed braver than most. A fine fellow should be rewarded with small pieces of cheese to take from my hand.

The mornings grew darker and journeys to Southampton in the winter months through rain, sleet, snow, and fog were cold, dark, and bleak. However, when I returned from the treatment there was little robin by the gate waiting for me.

Almost to the day as the radiotherapy finished, my friend flew away. I like to think that he knew I did not need him anymore, and now that it was the spring it was time for him to look after a family of his own.

The nurse walked across to my chair. I could tell by the smirk on her face she was about to answer my blood type query.

"Well Jacqueline, your blood type, believe it or not, is B POSITIVE. All I can say is that this certainly mirrors your attitude and positive personality." She grinned at Jacquie and me and then checked how the saline flush was going.

"We're nearly done, just a few more minutes and then we can get you on your way".

Jacquie looked at me shaking her head chuckling. "Well," she said looking a bit smug about it, "I guess it just had to be, really". How uncanny, this did just about sum up my attitude with all this rubbish going on.

Once I was "off the hook" we made our way to my local bar in Shirley, called Santo Lounge. It is a chain of bars which are open all day for breakfast right through until late night closing. We decided to order two glasses of Prosecco. The manager asked what the special occasion was, and we both looked at her smiling and I said, "getting through my second round of chemo treatment". The manager smiled, made our drinks, and turned around to place our glasses on the bar.

"These are on the house ladies, well done and keep positive." We thanked her and then took our seats away from the bar to chill and have some together time before Jacquie had to drop me back to my flat and head all the way back to Birmingham.

The discomfort I felt in my body up until the first treatment had begun to subside once my second chemotherapy started to kick in. I noticed a difference in my stomach and the way I was feeling. The changes continued to vary throughout my cycles, and I sometimes suffered with indigestion, sometimes very sore mouth ulcers and a few headaches.

Later in the month I was back at the hospital with Dr Green to discuss my bloods. My CA125 bloods started at eight hundred and sixty and went down to four hundred, so dropping by half, which was expected by the medical team. Then after the second treatment they had miraculously dropped to one hundred and eighty-one. The medical team were made up with these results to see how quickly the treatment was working to shrink the cancer in my body. Never did they expect another big drop like this. Happy days! I might still suffer some affliction but knowing the treatment was proving successful made it all worth it.

My current worry was now with my finances. I was not breaking the bank, but I also was not flush with money. I lived comfortably, yet my worry was about the time off work, the reduction in pay I could receive, the worry of a job loss if this was prolonged, losing my home and independence, and the time it would take me to get back onto the saving ladder and build up my money again. Just so many worries in my head that I needed to get them ironed out.

I made an appointment to speak to a member of the team at the Macmillan Centre to get financial advice. They got me in within two days. I spoke with a lady called Eve about my financial circumstances and she went through the appropriate forms with me to see if there was any way we could reduce my payments in any areas of my budget.

This is one of many services Macmillan provide for cancer patients and talking such worries over with a professional is taking away some of that extra stress you don't need whilst you are in this cancer bubble.

Tidying up financial details such as things like car finance monthly payments, etc can take a load off your mind. Macmillan also look at any benefits certain people might be able to apply for depending on their individual circumstances.

Although I still had some work to do on this, just going there to talk and straighten everything out in my mind had made me feel better about things. Later that day my cousin Liz and I took a big bunch of flowers to my auntie Brenda and spent the afternoon with her nattering over a nice cuppa. I appreciate my precious family time, always so much to talk about and so much laughter. It makes me completely forget about what is going on in the background and relieves me of the stress and worry of it all.

* * *

Chapter Nine

Cake, Benali, and the Great South Run

Last week of September, and Chemo Day had arrived again. My skin felt slightly itchy that morning. I knew it was probably the chemo reacting in my body. My face felt sensitive, warm and tingly, and I could feel the occasional aching around my kidneys – a reminder to keep up my water intake.

Fiona came with me again and this time we were told there was no room in the main treatment areas and the hospital might have to defer the chemo by a day or two or they might be able to give me my own room. This worried me straight away as I didn't want to be turned away so early on in my treatment. They asked Fiona and me to wait whilst they sorted this out for me. A lady called Lorraine took control for us, and she managed to get us in.

"Come with me ladies, we're upgrading you to your own room for the day; you'll be having your treatment in one of the upstairs suites."

Fiona looked at me and we both smirked smugly at each other. We followed Lorraine upstairs to get settled for the day with poor Fi acting as my entourage with what seemed like 50 bags!!! Me, the typical bag lady who never travelled light. Well, being a comfort girl, I didn't want the worry of what I might need as opposed to having everything I could with me just in case!

The day after I was feeling quite tired, and this feeling stayed with me for a couple of days. When my parents popped in to see me, I could tell they noticed this in me. I continued to rest up, drink fluids to stay hydrated and get as much sleep on and off as I possibly could. I dealt with the nausea and rode through the whiting out feelings as best I could. Spots appeared on my head for which I had nothing in the flat but antiseptic cream to use. I applied this very sparingly and it seemed to help.

I was experiencing some twinging in my ovary area, just about where I thought the large tumours were situated. Maybe this was the feeling you get when your tumours are beginning to shrink. These twinges came and went in waves. They were not painful, more like spasms.

As the days went by, I continued to eat healthily and started applying the antiseptic cream to my face where it was becoming slightly spotty. Another reaction, and I was sure there would be many more body changes still to come.

I guess the only way to describe how I felt about my appearance was to say my body changes resembled something like the effects of drinking Polyjuice from a Harry Potter movie. To others the changes during my treatment were probably not that noticeable, apart from my balding head. They all still saw me as me but, I saw my changes and didn't like them, yet what else could I do but get on with it?

This was just the way I was feeling as in time my body became bloated from the steroids, itchy and spotty skin, and cuts not healing as quickly as normal. Others going through this could feel differently about their looks or not even care, as the main point of all this is to try and stay alive. There will be people out there who will feel like they are changing into someone they don't know both in their looks and in their personality.

Such feelings can really knock a person's confidence at the best of times, let alone during illness and treatment. I feel it is so important to tell people they are not alone. Even if you can't talk about how you're feeling to friends and family, then visit or call a local charity who will talk to you and be more than understanding about what you are going through.

It was nearing time for the Macmillan Coffee Morning, for which my friend Carrie had organised to hold a cake baking day at her home in my honour. This was such a kind gesture and something else for me to look forward to. It's a yearly event held across the country to raise money for the Macmillan charity and usually falls at the end of September.

I suffered headaches all morning but put this down to the fact I was a tad excited about getting together with everyone to eat cake and donate! I arrived with my pre-baked goodies including sausage, apple and bacon filo pastries and was feeling in a cheerful mood.

Carrie was carrying her second child, Joe, and her little girl Lily was waiting around the table for the fun and cake to begin. The rest of the girls arrived with their baked goods and my cousin balancing her cakes in one hand and baby carrier in the other with new-born Alegria, named after a character in Cirque Du Soleil. We had a wonderful afternoon chatting, drinking tea, eating cakes, and enjoying cuddles with the kiddies. Holding a coffee morning for someone brings people together to spend time with each other, talking of our experiences and sharing our stories and supporting each other. These Macmillan events are so important for those affected, be it the person with the illness or their loved ones. Between us all we polished off a few naughty treats and raised money at the same time for a great cause.

Anyone who can make the effort to give just a little of their time to someone is so important and precious. It is great to have people to turn to, offering to drive you places, help to do your shopping, go for walks or coffee. It is often the little things in life we take for granted, which a person struggling with an illness will feel is making a world of difference. Such gestures alleviate the worry and stress and take away that feeling of helplessness.

I am lucky enough to have a good network of friends, as well as my entire family and throughout this whole ordeal I had waves of visitors to hospital, people offering regularly to take me out, do my shopping, have me stay over or cook me dinner. The support I had was unbelievable. I knew people cared but I didn't realise just how something like this could affect those so much in my life. A couple of times I have heard people say, "you reap what you sow", or "you often do so much for others, and now it's your turn". I have never been someone in life who gives to receive; however, it is nice that people wanted to help me in my time of need.

I have learned a lot since my illness, and I have come to realise who has been there for me most and those who were not. I feel that cancer can scare off people who have been affected in their own life by illness or death, and they probably find it hard to cope with such news, and therefore gave me a wide birth. Maybe for some, they can only just about deal with their own lives and stresses, and probably have no room mentally to take on something this challenging and upsetting. It is probably easier for them to cushion their own feelings rather than be there for me in the worry they may show them outwardly. I know I have been guilty of this in my past for fear of being a blubbering mess.

Sometimes when I think of my brush with death, it hurts my feelings that I had a lack of support from a minority of those I considered close to me. It took me a while to come to terms with this, but I knew if I wanted to keep these friendships I had to snap out of that mindset, draw a line under it and move on, otherwise resentment can sink in and it can fester if you don't deal with your feelings at the time it happens. I keep telling myself that not every individual reacts the same way. Not everyone in life will reciprocate a friendship or relationship in the same way and just because I might feel close to some people doesn't always mean that they should be the ones there at the front of the queue to support me.

My support network knows who they are, I do not have to tell them, they just know. They supported me day in and day out, and nothing has ever been too much trouble for them. I think as we get older our relationships with people do change and this whole cancer experience has taught me a lot about my different friendships and my feelings. I deal with stuff differently now. I do not have the same tolerance anymore for people who constantly moan about trivial stuff, and I don't worry anymore if someone doesn't have the time for me. I get on with life doing what makes me happy and with those who want to share it with me. My illness is slowly changing my perspective on things and what is important for me. I refrain from doing things just to please others. I am now the key person that I should be thinking about first. That is where my priorities lay as I continued to move forwards on my journey and lead a more balanced lifestyle and stay stress-free and happy.

October appeared and I was still suffering with my mouth ulcers and some chest pain. There was twinging pain to my right ovary area and this was also apparent in my right leg. The spasms felt like a minor electrical shock deep within, that caught me off guard and made me flinch. When I called the Macmillan nurses to discuss this, they reassured me this was quite a normal thing to be feeling.

I brushed this aside and kept focused on doing all the right things to keep my body strong. I went for my CT scan to check my chest, as well as my abdomen and pelvis. I knew the multi-disciplinary team were meeting the following day to discuss me, so I kept busy around all this with seeing people and being treated to lots of nice surprises – I guess my illness had its uses!

My cousin Sarah came with me to my next chemo session. I kept her occupied with my many demands and she kept me well entertained with her humour. I packed not just for the day, but so I could go spend a few days with Sarah and her family after my ordeal.

We arrived in plenty of time and the nurse took us round to get us settled in ready to undergo another unwanted but much needed cancer-killing drug dosage. Whilst there the hospital team advised me that my hysterectomy surgery date would be booked within 4 weeks and thereafter, I would be having two more cycles, 5 and 6, to zap any microscopic seedlings that could be floating. The team said my hair loss would be very drug dependant.

Whilst recouping with my cousins for a few days, I noticed that my ovary area was twinging a lot more frequently. I believed the chemo must be working its magic on me and so I continued to BELIEVE. Mainly because I had set myself a goal to be well enough for a big charity event taking place on the Sunday and I wanted to be there to photograph it, because it involved another one of life's big inspirations; Francis Benali.

Francis Benali is a former Southampton Football Club player. He regularly raises awareness and money running and cycling in aid of the Cancer Research charity. My family and I went along to the next estate from where they lived. There were many supporters waiting along the planned route to cheer Francis on.

I wanted to be a part, of what was to me, a very poignant event, playing a supporting role with the community in a great moment in time, whilst capturing photos of Francis and his entourage of runners there by his side.

Such a selfless person he is, with the strength and determination to make a difference to people living with cancer. It is people like him who have given me the fight and determination to take my journal a step further in writing this book, in the hope it will also help and encourage others as he has done.

Francis's ultra-challenge started at the beginning of October to visit all 44 premier league football stadiums within 2 weeks. Francis's challenge saw him running a marathon and cycling 75 miles each day. He had a huge fan support along the way and during his run, several of his family members, including his son, friends, and some famous faces, joined in on different dates to be with Francis and encourage him.

What with cash buckets being filled along his route, and Francis's donation webpage, it was reported that he ended up raising over £350,000 for Cancer Research, and probably a lot more thereafter. What an achievement!

The man did well, considering the agonising pain he endured throughout it all. This event was later televised on TV, showing the public just how much heart and soul Francis put into it with his team. He seems such a humble, down to earth person. He is a family man who uses his status to do good in this world with the help of many other famous TV personalities. He has a big heart and is a true hero in my eyes.

Suddenly my brother's birthday had crept up on me. I had not purchased a gift in time due to my mind being on the chemo side of things, and my little jolly out to photograph Benali and Co had taken the wind out of me. I wasn't feeling well enough to drive just under a two-hour journey to his hometown of Weymouth. I purchased a voucher and card and called him to say I would be sending him something in the post as this was the easier thing for me to do at this time.

Tony's answer to me … "the greatest gift for me is knowing you are still here in my life". Gosh, the things people say that just touch your heart and fill you with emotion. God love him.

My brother was not concerned about material things. He wanted me better and he knew the best way for me to do this was to try baby steps first without exerting myself too much to help get myself back into a normal life pattern. He knew I had to rest after the Benali event as I was still experiencing the twinging pangs in my stomach.

I was in hospital with my surgeon to sign off my Patient Agreement paperwork for investigation and treatment of a hysterectomy and omentectomy. Mr Hadwin was happy with how my body had been responding to treatment and happy that we would be going ahead with my operation in November.

"Jackie, we will be doing a total debulking operation of the omentum, uterus, neck of cervix, tubes with ovaries, and other tumours. Thereafter the cells will be microscopically tested, the team can then review the type of cell behaviour and will be able to explain what the cells are doing."

"Can you explain how the operation is going to happen please?"

"Yes, we will be looking to cut vertically from your lower tummy up as far as your belly button to open the stomach cavity to see better when exploring around. "

'Bloody-hell, this sounds like a jungle expedition, not an operation,' I thought.

"Should any further spread of cancer be found during this procedure, then there is a possibility we will cut up to your chest if necessary. Jackie this is going to be a major operation. Your skin and fat layers will be cut into, and there could be a risk of injury to the bowel and bladder."

Next, I was shown to another room with two nurses to go through my pre-op prep and take away with me a surgical body wash to use a few days leading up to and after my operation. Nose and groin swabs were done and then my blood pressure taken.

Then as we sat chatting and my verbal mouth gates opened once again with questions. They just keep pouring out like the rapid waters of the Niagara Falls. I am inquisitive and each time I got an answer, it prompted another question and so on. I seem to be asking anything and everything and probably outdid the Encyclopaedia Britannica with the knowledge I gained. I wanted to know, good or bad; I needed to know what I was walking in to. Some people prefer not to know; they just want the cancer gone and to get back to a normal life, and that is okay too.

The nurses talked through my operation process. They said a spinal injection would be done locally to the site and numb the nerves for around four or five hours. A spinal is good for pain relief and for the gut after surgery. The injection would be put into the surrounding sac and there can be nerve damage to the tissues and some feeling can be lost.

"Jackie you may experience headaches afterwards. However, the nurses attend regularly to give pain relief and other drugs. If you read, then bring glasses and reading books to surgery. We'll have a plan for the day and won't know until then which order patients will be taken down to theatre.

The nurse explained the outer body tissue would take approximately two weeks to heal and I needed to keep this covered and dry during this time. Then it would take up to eight weeks for the inside healing. After this time, I could look to start driving again. Most people spend around three to five days in hospital. "You will be monitored each day and see how you are progressing, and once we feel you are moving about on your legs and your bowel movements are OK then you will be discharged to go home. Please ensure you arrange with friends or family about emergency contact numbers as we will need this information when you are admitted for surgery."

I asked if I could climb upstairs straight away, and they told me I would be encouraged to get up and move about as soon as possible to ensure blood circulation around the body to prevent clotting.

"So, just to recap, Jackie. Your recovery will take up eight weeks in total. During this time, you should not do any lifting, no driving, ensure you get up and out of bed and move about but also balance this with a lot of good rest and sleep. Keep up your fluids, so drink plenty of water. Increase your walking distance gradually and with what you are comfortable with. Your post-op follow-up will be approximately two weeks after surgery then chemotherapy will start after this. Post-op you will need to contact your Macmillan team for any further help and advice. The operation can make you menopausal; however, this is something you will discuss later at future clinics."

I was glad to get this out the way as my next journey was to Portsmouth on the 23rd to photograph the Great South Run. This is a big event held yearly which covers a flat running course past many landmarks including the Spinnaker Tower, Portsmouth's Historic Dockyard (past Nelson's flagship the HMS Victory) and Southsea Seafront to round it off to the finish line.

Iwan Thomas was present at this event and was running for Macmillan Cancer Charity. Iwan is a British sprinter and has represented Great Britain and Northern Island at the Olympic Games and Wales for the Commonwealth Games. He has worked on many a TV show.

He is involved in many local races and charity events, and for the Great South Run Iwan's chosen charity was the Macmillan Cancer Charity. He, along with many well-known TV personalities, are involved in many local charity events and he spends time at the starting line for press coverage and to talk to the people who turn out to watch and to encourage all the runners taking part. I'd noticed him there since I started photographing this event for Macmillan a few years ago, way before I was even diagnosed with my illness.

He also shows such great support for local sporting events as well as large, televised events that take place across the country. Iwan loves to contribute to the community spirit and engaging with the public. He is another great personality and a particularly good role model for young people.

My brother Tony has run various races in the past of which the London Marathon and the Great South Run for Macmillan are two of them, so he is no stranger to this course. His leg was damaged in the lead up to the race and he struggled on the day. As he was about two thirds round, he began to slow his running pace and then this became more of a brisk walk then on to a kind of hobbling along. Tony admitted he found this race a struggle but continued to hobble slowly round the track in front of hundreds of supporters. Next thing Tony felt something on his shoulder. It was another runner in the race giving my brother some encouragement. This spurred my brother on to get his mojo back and pick up his pace again to get round the race and over that finish line in my honour and for Macmillan.

Although I admire all who ran and I am inspired by the TV personalities who attend, in my eyes there were two main stars that day. The man with his encouraging words and my brother for finding the strength in battling through his pain to reach that finish line.

Not only has the Great South Run become another yearly ritual of mine to go photograph, but also for those in my family. For years we have run for different cancer charities to help raise money and awareness. My cousins ran the Great South Run with my brother the following year and although they ran it many times before, this one was in my honour for Macmillan. My cousin Dan had not long recovered from brain surgery. It was devastating to think we could have lost him, yet he was nearing his recovery and there at the start line, standing ready to run ten long miles amongst the thousands of runners taking part. I felt such a sense of pride and emotion. It made me think of what strength we have just within our family. For Dan to do this for me just speaks volumes and this touched my heart in a big way. He is such a caring and selfless human being. Over the years we have all entered charity races, long before my cancer diagnosis but, I guess it all seems much more important to me now.

Next, another routine check-up pre-chemo with my friend Karen. These clinics are an ongoing process to see how I am feeling, what my body has been doing or not doing and just have a general chat about my health. I self-check in and take a ticket from the machine. It is like being at the deli counter in a supermarket, but instead of waiting my turn for a wedge of cheese or a succulent cut of meat, I am waiting for my number to be called to get weighed and give bloods! Once done at the "deli" I am called through for my routine chat to discuss how my bloods are still doing.

Dr Green never knows what I am going to walk in with as I do not sit quietly for too long, and I always seem to collate a long list of questions from my ongoing research ready for when I see her. She must think she is the one being interviewed at times. All seemed to still be heading in the right direction and both Dr Green and the Macmillan nurses were amazed with my progress and the fact my bloods had taken a fast-descent right down to a mere 6. It was incredible what my body was doing, and the medical team were just as ecstatic as I was with this outcome. A few days after this I endured my last chemo session before my operation date.

* * *

Chapter Ten

And Breathe......

Between the dates of November 9th and 12th, I experienced a sense of anxiety about my op, and I seemed doubtful this was going to be a good outcome. I had been a little tense as I also knew how much this was affecting my family and close friends. I was praying we could rid of this cancer, and even though I always see the positive in a bad situation, I still had my doubts about what the outcome would be. I think this is because of the many people I know who have been through similar cancer experiences, some of whom are still with us and those who lost their lives too early to this.

My cousin Jane booked up a spa session so that I could go and take things easy and forget about it all for a short while. During this I was mindful not to use any of the pool, jacuzzi or steam room facilities due to possible cross contamination. This was advised by the hospital just in case I did have any open wounds or pierced skin made during hospital blood tests that could get infected.

I telephoned ahead to enquire about massage treatments. It was recommended I went with a massage for pregnant ladies due to my condition and they would only treat me on the basis I got a letter from the hospital explaining what I could have done. Although I was not able to make use of all the pool & jacuzzi facilities, this was a treat, so I wanted to ensure I made the most of the day. I packed a holdall so I could entertain myself and stick to doing the simpler things there. I took my flip flops to keep my feet protected when walking around the spa and pool areas, a good reading book and some magazines. I sat by the pool reading and relaxing while my cousin took to the pool to swim a few lengths. After a while, she got out and we took a walk round to one of the quiet rooms. We stepped inside the room and got ourselves comfortable on the empty loungers positioned across the room from each other. The warm orange glow of the ambient light already set the mood for a lazy, chilled afternoon. Playing in the background I heard gentle windchimes like spiritual sounding music. My senses took a hold, and I noticed a subtle smell of aromatherapy fragrance in the room, which I found very relaxing and gave me an instant urge of wanting to sleep.

We probably talked for what seemed like seconds before closing our eyes. I felt myself starting to breathe slowly and deeply, inhaling, and exhaling the earthy scent in the room. It smelt a bit like sandalwood and once I got the breathing going, I started to feel as though I was beginning to float, and the weight I had been carrying dissolved. This room was awesome, and the whole experience was just what my body needed. This gift was a perfect "to do" day together to just to go chat, chill and forget about everything else that had been going on in Jackie's hectic little world.

I think if a spa is what someone going through cancer wants to do, then it is better to prep prior to the spa day by making a call ahead to speak to someone who is qualified. By giving the therapists pre-warning, they advised the best treatments tailored to me, thus helping to keep me safe from any contraindications. This saves a lot of time on the day and the possibility of being refused treatment.

Most establishments will ask up front for you to bring along a letter from the hospital. This is because your health is paramount and covers them as a business. Planning will ensure everything is done safely and above board and you feel comfortable throughout. I think a spa experience should be a fulfilling one, and give you a feeling of calm and relaxation.

I sought to download a meditation app to my phone and found this particularly useful indeed. Especially at night when I would get settled into bed, and my mind began to wonder endlessly about everything.

There are many different apps for all kinds of things so always try a few out to see which you are best suited to. The one I stuck to and still use today is called Insight Timer. It has many varied meditation sessions at different time settings. They have a wide choice of music, instrumental pieces, voices counting you into sleep and nature sounds. It is about finding what is right for you in aiding you to have some calm in your routine to give your body and mind a break and let go.

* * *

Chapter Eleven

Under the Knife

My pre-op assessment took place on Wednesday November 9th, 2016, and then I was scheduled to have the full hysterectomy on the following Tuesday. In the week leading up to this operation I started to feel very anxious and doubtful about the outcome of it all. It was just nerves kicking in a bit as I had never gone through major surgery before, and I realised this was also a big thing for my family to have to endure.

The nurse took me to a room to go through my pre-op instructions about what I could and could not eat/drink before the operation and to discuss my current medications. I was asked to give a urine sample and she checked me over. We spoke of my admission plan and then she gave me a bottle of pre-op Hibiscrub anti-bacterial wash to use and some pre-op drinks to take on the evening before my operation, and again the next day along with some yellow pills. Even though I was given a pamphlet on what to do, I listened intently as it all seemed to be so much to take in.

Due to the expansion of my now tight stomach, my belly button was feeling very sore and uncomfortable. I just wanted this all to be over and to have recovered within a few weeks so I could get back to my job and have some routine again.

November 15th and operation Jackie was about to commence.

Bag at the ready with my essentials. Although it may seem obvious to most what to pack for a hospital visit, knowing what I know now,

I just say pack anything that is a home comfort for you and will keep you occupied during your hospital time. My added reference pages are purely suggestions based on my own personal experiences and what I felt I needed for my situation.

See reference pages at back of this book

This operation was a major one. It was carried out to remove the cancer and do a full hysterectomy on me. We had an early start as my operation was scheduled for 07.45. My parents and brother came with me.

We arrived early at the hospital and were advised to sit in the relatives waiting room outside the Day Unit. I could tell from my parents and brothers' behaviour that they were trying to be upbeat and chatty to pass the time, but I could also read their faces and feel their pain. I hated the fact I was trying to be brave for them, yet they were slowly cracking inside and still trying to stay as upbeat as possible. There was another family sat just across the room from us. I don't know why they were there or who was having an op carried out. It was a tense time and the four of us just spoke amongst ourselves.

A nurse popped by and asked me to follow her to get gowned up and then I could come back round to my family and wait until I was called through for my surgery. I was taken through to a waiting area with a few empty beds with chairs beside each one. A curtain was drawn around me and the nurse asked me to slip out of my clothing and into a gown and to put on the white knee length support socks provided. These were used to help prevent blood clotting during and after my operation. I then had bloods and my blood pressure taken. "Mr Hadwin will be round shortly to speak to you and then you can go back to the family waiting area".

I sat reading my book with my sexy stockings on, no makeup, no hair, no eyelashes, no underwear under my gown. I felt totally stripped of everything, just there in a gown waiting to be put on the slab ready to be dissected, like the rat in biology class at school. I remembered that

116

class because we were doing something completely out of my comfort zone. I remember cutting too far down the rat's stomach with my knife and looking down in shock at a kind of dangly bit with what looked like a gland with tiny veins attached to it. To this day I still don't know if I had cut that poor little rat's willy, testicles or what off! Funny the things that pop into your head when you start over thinking or worry about something. My brain always worked overtime and normally at the wrong times!

Mr Hadwin stepped around the curtain and took a pew on the bed to talk to me.

He went through all my paperwork to ensure I understood the full internal debulking procedure and the risks involved with infections and blood clotting.

"There may be a slight tingling to the hands and feet which can persist after treatment, and although there are hard nodules in the peritoneal lining, the debulking surgery may include removing part of the bowel."

Mr Hadwin continued with asking me further questions and checking my details. We finished up, I signed the necessary paperwork, then I went back to the waiting room with my family.

Again, sitting tentatively waiting for that dreaded moment when I would be taken from them. It is harder to deal with something like this when you are sitting there knowing how your loved ones must be feeling. I knew it was a major op, but I had never had a major op before, so my worry was mainly about their feelings and how they were trying to cope.

In walked a nurse and called my name. She said for me to follow her through once I was ready to do so. It was time. I got up to say my temporary goodbyes and hugged my dad, my brother, and my mum each in turn. My heart was racing but I knew this would be the next step on my journey in helping me to get my life back. My family each held me tight, and I could feel my mum shaking as she started to break down in tears. It wasn't nice. In fact, it was bloody heart wrenching; however, I managed to compose myself as both my parents began to get upset.

I hate you cancer for what you are doing to my family.

I hate you cancer because in the past you took loved ones from me, far too soon.

I hate you cancer for causing so much hurt and pain to so many people in the world.

I hate you cancer because you kill and you have no good reason to be present.

Go do one cancer because I DON'T want you. You are intrusive and nasty, and you do not belong.

I turned to my brother and said, "Tony please make sure you look after mum and dad". To this day I am not sure why I asked that of my brother as he looked like he was on the verge of breaking point. What was I thinking? How could I possibly ask this of him when he was fighting the emotions back himself? It's times like this that prevent us from thinking straight and we can say the most bizarre things when in this state of mind.

I was being escorted back to my waiting bed. The nurse then asked me to get on the bed and within seconds of doing so, I was being wheeled down to theatre. There would be students in the room during my op which I had given my consent to. I remember a few people in the room talking and although I felt very anxious, I also felt at ease with them talking to me and telling me what they were doing.

A gentleman stood behind my head looking down at me.

"Hello Jacqueline, I'm your anaesthetist today and this is my team who will be helping me throughout the procedure."

A young female nurse then spoke, "I'm putting these pads on your arms and chest. These are to monitor your situation throughout the procedure."

The anaesthetist spoke again, "I am about to give you an injection. Once I've injected you, I will ask you to count down for me from five to one".

I remember laying there watching the people around me, doing their job, ensuring I was as comfortable as I could be, giving me words of encouragement and assuring me that I was in safe hands.

"Okay Jacqueline, we're ready now, and I would like you to start counting down for me." I said nothing and just nodded at him then counted, "five, four, three" ... bang. Out like a light.

* * *

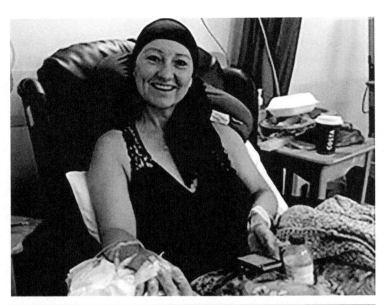

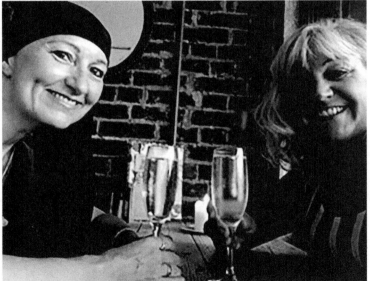

Top: *My 2nd Chemo*
Bottom: *A post-chemo drink with Jacquie as a way of sticking our fingers up to cancer*

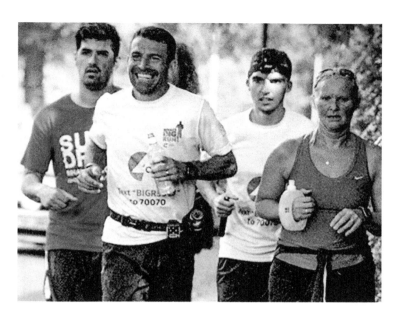

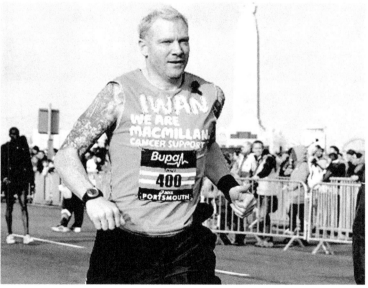

Francis Benali (Top) and Iwan Thomas (Bottom) who with their constant charity events continue to raise awareness and money for cancer.

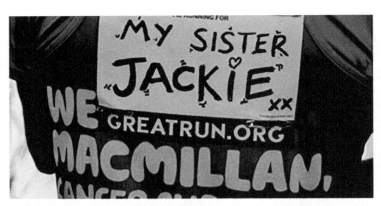

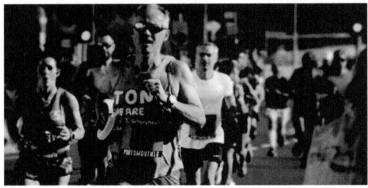

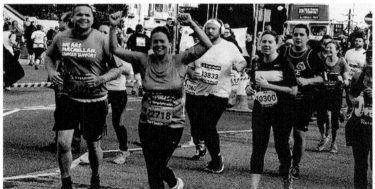

My cousins Sarah and Dan and my brother Tony running the Great South Run for Macmillan. Dan had not long had surgery, yet he still supported me.

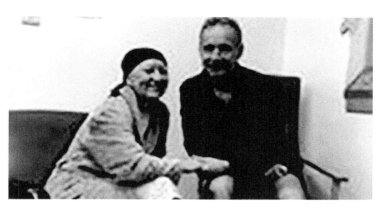

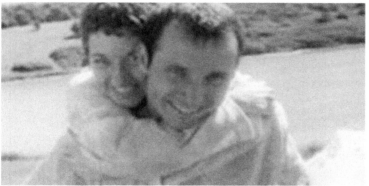

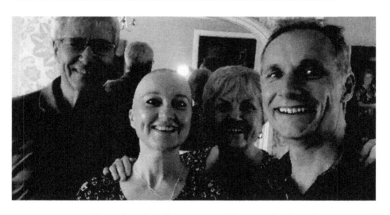

My parents and my brother keep me smiling with their humour and unconditional love

Chapter Twelve

Sledgehammer

"Jacqueline, Jacqueline, can you hear me? How are you doing?" I could hear this soft voice, but everything seemed dark for a short while as if I was dreaming. I then realised this was no dream, and it was the nurse gently talking to me as I started to slowly come round.

I don't think I had taken into consideration just how big a procedure this was, and to think I was the one consoling everyone prior to my operation and telling them it would be OK. Upon waking up, I felt like I had been hit tenfold with a sledgehammer. The pain was unbelievably excruciating. I felt tired and groggy which was fully to be expected, yet I hadn't thought I would wake up and feel like I had been bashed to a complete pulp! I doubt Mike Tyson could have done a better job on me if he tried. I shifted slightly and OMG! The pain!

Realisation was now really starting to sink in. I lay there in shock at the traumatic feeling in my body and in disbelief that I had thought I was going to come round from this in an 'okay' state.

The nurse smiled at me. "Can I sit you up for a bit Jacqueline? I'll help you and we'll take it slowly". *My god, I thought, seriously, how does this woman expect me to try to sit up in this much pain? Surely, she's not going to just hoist me up into position like right now, surely not! She can't be!* The nurse clocked my facial expression of complete surprise and shock at her request.

"Don't worry, we'll do this in your own time, just let me know when you are ready, and we'll start."

Yep! She bloody well was going to get me up, right this minute.

"Okay Jacqueline, I'm going to use this remote control on the side of your bed first to bring you up so far and then on the count of three I'll help to pull you up and get you more comfortable."

Did she not think that I was quite comfortable enough where I was laying (within reason), rather than to interrupt me and my outrageously painful insides, just to move me to another position? 'This is going to be bloody awful', I thought. The nurse made her way around my bedside to start the remote control. *This is going to hurt like hell.* The nurse started to remotely position the bed up at about a forty-degree angle, although it felt like three-hundred and sixty degrees with the pain I was suffering. I felt my entire body break out in a sweat and for a split second thought my mouth was going to shout some rather profound obscenities. Before the big hoist began. I braced myself and took a silent deep breath.

"Okay Jacqueline are you ready?"

"Not really but go for it."

The nurse took my arm in hers, "here we go ... 1, 2, 3 okay, that's it, easy".

I looked at her, "are we done?"

"No, just one more to get you sitting comfortably."

Comfortably? Was she having a bloody laugh because I was not finding this at all comfortable?

I have a high pain threshold, and this must be the second most painful experience so far in the whole hospital process for sure. First the biopsy and now this. At least with the biopsy it was all done and dusted whereas this pain I had now I think was going to be with me for quite a few weeks to come.

I was given some pain killers, a blood thinner injection to my stomach called Clexane, and had my blood pressure tested and temperature taken.

"Would you like me to bring you a cup of tea Jacqueline?"

A cuppa? Now that was music to my ears. No matter what blows in life you take, you can always guarantee on a nice cuppa to make things feel a little bit better.

I looked around the ward to see three other women who were each in for different operations. We all made small talk in between reading our books and having visits from the nurses.

Visiting hours were starting later that day and I knew my wonderful family would be waiting impatiently in anticipation of getting to my bedside. I lay there feeling broken and still in shock from the sheer pain, and then there they were, my parents and brother all walking into the ward towards my bed. In that moment watching them all walk in behind one another, my anxiety dissolved, and the feeling of pain lifted for a short moment. I was so glad to see them, and I broke out in the biggest smile. It was the biggest relief for us all that I had come through. Although the drugs were still swimming around in my system and I was feeling a bit out of it, I could see the elation in their faces.

They took their seats around my bedside, and we chatted for a while about how I was feeling and what they had been doing to pass the time whilst I was having my op. Then my sense of humour kicked in.

"Tony, can you pass me that cardboard bed pan from over there please".

Tony gave me the bed pan thinking that I needed to use it and then I turned it upside down and placed it on my head like a trilby hat and asked Tony to take a photo of myself wearing it. I pulled a stupid face as he took the shot. We all laughed about it at the time but, now when I look at that picture, it makes me realise just how sick I looked, and how unlike me it looked. I don't think I realised the full extent of just how serious this all was from their perspective. Or maybe it was that I chose to live life and keep strong for all those around me who were crumbling, or worried for me.

I should have been going home within a day or two; however, I was in hospital for six days. That meant six days of stomach injections, six days of popping pills, six days of having my bloods and blood pressure taken, six days of nurses encouraging me to get up and walk, five restless nights of feeling cold and trying to sleep in the thinnest of bed sheets and blankets I'd ever seen, and six days of watching a wave of patients coming in, and out of my ward after their operations after getting the thumbs up they could go home.

Me? – Well, it was obvious I was not going anywhere until they felt I was able to move my bowels. The pain of the operation was bad, so goodness knows how I was going to feel when I eventually had to go! Having to get up and walk about to exercise whilst still in gut wrenching pain had to be the third most excruciating pain that I endured during my hospital treatment. It was such intense pain when I tried to make any kind of movement, sit up or get out of bed. It was a feeling like no other, and ironically, as if my insides had been aggressively ripped out of me.

The thing with an operation like this, is that straight away the nurses have you up and out of bed on the first day after surgery. This is to keep the blood circulation moving and help reduce the risks of any complications developing, such as blood clots in your legs. I thought I was dying inside and so scared my bloody insides were going to rip open or fall out of my vagina!! I know people who have had a normal hysterectomy (without having all the cancer removed with secondary procedures), who had pre-warned me of the pain but, no matter how many times someone said that to me, it didn't sink in until I woke up from it all … then the nightmare began. It was to be six days of sheer and utter pain and no escape.

Kerry came to spend some time up at the hospital with me, which was a big comfort and helped me forget the pain I was in for a while. I saw the shock in her face straight away and knew because of her experience with her auntie that it probably felt like she was reliving it all. Kerry is a strong person with a tough exterior, but this had hit her hard - something she didn't confess to me until months later. It was during this discussion she admitted she had never seen me looking so pale and lifeless and it really upset her.

The hospital was keeping a close eye on me and said that once they were happy that my bowels were back in working order I could go home. Each day I prayed it would be the day I had a poo, so I could get out of the ward and be more comfortable at home with my family.

The duty nurse popped into the ward one evening to give me a Clexane injection. She talked me through the process as she was showing me how to inject my stomach and said I would be taking home a box of these to inject myself with around the same time every evening for a month.

"You can either have someone do this for you, or you can do it yourself."

"Myself?!"

"Yes. I'll pop in at the same time tomorrow evening and you can have a go at doing this yourself."

She explained this injection was to thin my blood to reduce the risk of blood clots by stopping them from forming. Upon being discharged from hospital, they would give me my prescription drugs and Clexane injections, along with a sharps box to put them in after use.

Discharge date from the Bramshaw Women's Unit: Sunday 20th November 2016.

I was given a discharge summary of the operation that had taken place for my records. It stated in the summary that the whole procedure was a gynae operation which included a primary procedure of a total abdominal hysterectomy. This was the removal of the uterus, cervix, fallopian tubes etc. On top of that they did two secondary operations. One was to remove both of my ovaries, called a bilateral oophorectomy and the other, omentectomy, was to remove part or all, of the abdominal lining. The tissue of the omentectomy procedure is called the omentum. It is a fatty organ and is made up of an area of lining called the peritoneum. The peritoneum encases the stomach and other abdominal organs.

I would be given a scan around mid-February to check how everything had settled down.

HRT was mentioned again by the hospital this time. It was recommended to help my heart and bones – due to calcium and vitamin D deficiencies. However, I strongly felt this was something I wanted to deal with on my own and then if I suffered with the early menopause kicking in, I would re-consider my options.

I had more questions about exercises, when the dressing should come off, how long to wear the hospital stockings, etc.

Whilst waiting for the nurses to prep my post-op meds and sign off my discharge papers so I could leave, I thought about a few things that had happened over the past few months. I learned that you need to be prepared for certain things that you may not be told by the hospital. They have so much to deal with and each patient will have a different hospital experience.

I then started to think about my brother and how heartbroken mum was to see him visit me and look at me in the state I woke up in. As we said our goodbyes mum had stood watching Tony from the hospital window walking back to his car, probably worrying himself sick about me, and then having to drive back down to Weymouth alone. I also remembered the nurse coming to get me to take me to surgery for my operation and me turning to Tony asking him to be strong for my parents.

I hate the fact I put so much pressure on my brother. It made me feel selfish that I was more concerned for how this was affecting my parents at their age and that I assumed that my brother would cope. I cannot believe that I asked that of him. What was I thinking? I know he is a strong person, but I know deep down how this would have affected me if the boot was on the other foot. I would have been devastated.

I now needed to keep focused on getting well and for our family to be happy. I was determined to get myself better but, I also knew this was going to be a long and painful road to recovery. I had come this far, so I wasn't going to stop at that point.

My friend, Claire, came to visit me that evening at my parent's home to see how I was doing. She stayed for a while chatting, and it was nice to catch up with her. I could feel the tiredness kicking in and my eyes becoming heavier. For a moment I was fighting it, but Claire could see this and after a good while with me she decided to make her move. When I look back at the post-op selfies I took whilst in hospital my face looks so sickly, pale, and bloated from the steroids. Goodness knows how I must have looked to Claire, and to many others who saw me around this time: death warmed up and a shell of what my healthier self once was, pre-cancer. The only other time I can think I probably looked my worst, or rather a complete mess, would be quite a few years back after a heavy night in town. We went to watch a gig at the Joiners pub, a place where grunge band, Nirvana, once played long before they made it big. Funnily enough, the two bands we watched that night were tribute bands called "Nearvana" and "The Foo Forgers". I drunkenly staggered straight out of that place and completely bulldozed it to the ground hitting my head on the curb. My friends felt sick at first because of the noise it made, but soon saw the funny side of it. We certainly knew how to raise the roof, and a bit too much sometimes. My single years have been well spent travelling and partying at gigs and festivals, and great memories lived with old friendships, and new ones made along the way.

It sounds silly but I often question things like my injuries and what I've put into my body over the years and if this had maybe somehow contributed to my outcome now. We read and hear so much through research, the news, magazine articles, etc about our bodies having precancerous cells that could turn cancerous in the right environment. This makes me question that just maybe I gave myself the match to ignite the cancer within me?

I stayed with my parents for the next couple of months to recover. The first couple of weeks I was in a lot of pain. It was more painful than I expected but still I was determined. I had to inject myself in my stomach area for twenty-four days after surgery with Clexane. I am not great with needles, so I need a medal for that one! To be honest, the needles were short, so if I managed to get through all my blood tests and cannulas being stuck in me regularly, then I had to just bite the bullet and do this one small thing each evening. I kept focusing on the end goal, NO CANCER.

The last week of November I experienced lots of painful wind movements and bleeding. I kept telling myself I had to endure all the pain to gain my life back.

My gang of girlies had been on a weekend away to the Cotswolds, which I should have joined them on. They had texted me as they wanted to come visit on route back home. I wasn't feeling up to it at all but they really wanted to pop by, and I knew this was because they care, and they would just spend a short time with me to cheer me up. I felt groggy and tired and found it difficult at times to keep my eyes open. My body was washed in waves of feeling hot and then getting a cold sweat and I felt as if I was going to be sick at times. Another text came from Fi to say they would just pop by for a moment and would not stay too long so as not to tire me out. However awful I felt, however much I didn't feel like seeing anyone, I didn't want to disappoint them, and I caved in, and they came by. It was great to see them and to hear about the fun they had had while away. As gutted as I was, I am glad they all enjoyed the weekend together. As usual, they showered me with gifts and goodies and then made their departure. My body felt completely done in and I slept for quite a while afterwards.

Beginning of December and the visits to the house from loved ones was still going strong. Many came bearing gifts and cards, and the odd bottle of wine ready for when I would be up to drinking.

I had removed my dressing on the hospital's advice, ready that week for when I had my clinic appointment. I had a lot of soreness around my tummy, my groin area and especially around the area I had been injecting. By the end of the month my sexy hospital stockings were peeled off.

I again had clinic. It all seemed to be a monotonous circle of appointments. This one was to catch up on my progress. We all talked of my blood type being B Positive and had another good giggle at that one. Questions were asked about me in general and I explained I was feeling okay mentally

I explained about the soreness after removing my dressing and that I had experienced uncomfortable spasms at night, but it had started slowing down as I was not feeling these spasms so much in the mornings now. My bowel movements were fine although to pass wind still hurt a lot, such a sharp pain but at least this meant it was all in working order. I told Dr Green that when peeing, it felt like my insides were going to drop out, and that I had underestimated the pain I would feel after surgery.

Dr Green advised me that whilst the surgeon had been working on me, he had found spots to my left fallopian tube and ovaries, but that nothing had to be lasered off my bowels. I was advised not to use swimming pools/spas due to picking up infections, and no massage treatments. My cervix was sewn over and would take six weeks to heal. I was to do pelvic floor exercises. The menopause would kick in immediately and I would get scans pre/post-my further chemo sessions. My clinic appointments would be monthly for a year, three monthly for two years and then six monthly after five years. My dental appointments could not be booked until three weeks after my last chemotherapy.

December 2016 saw one of my final two chemo sessions following on from my post-op recovery. Again, I went through the same procedures and made sure I got plenty of rest at home in between both sessions, as well as a few visits from friends and other relatives. I felt tired and sick but kept positive throughout. Only one more to go now.

* * *

Chapter Thirteen

Star Wars

Back in 2015 before I was ever diagnosed with cancer, Kerry's husband Darren had purchased cinema tickets for himself, his son Ethan, his father-in-law Stuart, and my good self (of course). Kerry was not a hard-core fan like us, so she left us all to our own devices.

We went to see The Force Awakens. There came that heart wrenching moment in the movie when Han Solo's character was killed off and I began to cry. It was like experiencing an end of an era for me because Star Wars is one of my childhood memories. Suddenly the tears stopped, and the embarrassment sunk in, when little Ethan laughed and spoke loudly enough for his dad to hear and many a movie goer sitting within hearing distance.

"Dad, dad, quick, look at Jackie". Ethan was still laughing at me, "she's crying dad, I knew she would cry if Han Solo got killed".

I looked across Darren and Stuart to where little Ethan was sitting, and the situation made us all smile. From that moment and throughout Christmas time, the smiles continued right through into the new year of 2016.

Another year on and our "Star Wars ritual day" was here. This was something I had really been looking forward to. How I contained my excitement is beyond me. Star Wars Rogue One, was showing at the Showcase Cinema in Southampton, and again I was there with the same crew.

It has become a yearly thing with us all to go and watch the new Star Wars movies together. Over the years, the new films have been screened around Christmas time, and then the occasional spin off films are shown during the year. The spin off films usually tells the story about a certain character or event from the main story lines and opens your heart and imagination to a whole new adventure into this sci-fi series.

As you can tell, I am a Star Wars buff, and have been since I was young. My dad took me and my brother to the cinema in nineteen eighty, just weeks after my tenth birthday, to see The Empire Strikes back. Although this was the second movie released, it was the first out of the original trilogy that I went to see at the cinema. This all came about because I kicked up such a big fuss at the time the first movie Star Wars – A New Hope was released. My dad arranged to take my brother and a couple of his friends in our street to see this one. At the time, I was not happy that they went to the cinema, and I was not included on the boys outing. In typical diva Jackie style, I threw all my toys out of the pram and thought life was so unfair and 'oh woe is me'.

I remember feeling chuffed to bits to be in the cinema watching the second movie, even though my brother still didn't class me as "one of the boys" I didn't care. I had got my own way this time and I was ready to watch the action and feel the excitement.

I warmed very quickly to the character, Han Solo. He was dashing and seemed to have a recklessness about him, like me. He was a cool character with a bad ass attitude, and a smile to die for. Over the years I grew to love a lot of the films Harrison Ford made outside of the Star Wars franchise. I could see what a versatile and amazing actor he was, and how much heart and soul he put into his movies. Harrison Ford is an inspiration to me because he works hard to get results and he gives so much joy to his audience.

After a nice festive break, there we were again, back in the hot seat. At least I had lots of Christmas leftovers to see me through this one! Jacquie was all the way back down from Bromsgrove to be with me. My parents turned up to literally spend a short time, stood talking with us. We discussed an idea I had for making some headbands. The idea came to mind because of the difficulties I had with trying to keep my scarves on.

"Maybe you should patent that idea Jackie and look into getting some made. Especially if you feel this will be beneficial to others".

Jac being a self-employed businesswoman discussed the possibilities and made me seriously consider it; however, you need money to make money and I didn't have that kind of outlay to put into starting this up. The time had come for my parents to leave the room and Jac and I to get on with our own devices. I gave them a massive hug and off they both trundled together out of sight.

By mid-January, my sixth chemo session was underway. It took me a while to combat the sickness feeling which the cocktail of chemo drugs gave me. I learned to gauge when I started to feel a bit of sickness coming on. I would sometimes feel a little warm before the nausea kicked in, so I would reach for some cold water. Occasionally I would eat something if I felt the need to, even if it was just a small bite of food to slowly chew on, or a sweet to suck on. Even now I find the water drinking a huge help in getting the sickness feeling to subside. My water bottle goes everywhere with me now.

All this helped rather than popping anti-sickness pills, which I tried to avoid taking too often. Every time I felt this way, I would drink more water which hydrated me and cooled me down somewhat. It seems to be the same principal as motion sickness, and it is learning how to combat this as you go.

Weeks after I had another CT Chest/Abdo/Pelvis scan at the hospital imaging suite. This was to check that all was well. My organs looked clear and there were no cheeky cancer seedlings partying in my belly.

February 10th, 2017 - my first day back to work on reduced hours. It was going to be a slow process reacquainting myself with staff in the building and the working environment. Slowly taking back parts of my workload bit by bit over time. I arrived outside and parked up in the car park and then pressed the intercom to gain entry to the building. My manager, Jo, was there to greet me back and we had a morning meeting scheduled to discuss a few things before starting the day. Upon opening the door to the reception area, I was filled with emotion to find my work area decorated with flowers, and a basket full of various healthy items. It was quite overwhelming, and I certainly felt the love.

My team are supportive, thoughtful, and generous. They do not do things because they feel they must; they do it because they care. It then dawned on me that they had all been here before with Alex. His illness got bad, and they lost him to cancer, and I suddenly realised everyone at my place of work had been reliving another cancer nightmare with me, not knowing if I would get better but always encouraging me with strong positive words and affection. Eventually we introduced me back to trying some full working days. However, much I needed to be back, it seemed a long day for me doing the whole eight hours, and so after the first full day I found myself driving to my friend Karen. When I had days where I struggled, I would often drive back to a friend's house for a cuppa to unwind and clear my mind - and often get a dinner cooked for me which was a result!

I had ongoing discussions with the hospital about what would happen once the Naraparib maintenance drugs were released on the market. I would then have my three monthly, six monthly and yearly check-ups whilst using the drugs. All seemed pretty clear and up front, and it was just a case of picking a suitable time and sticking to that time every day for the rest of my life or until such time as the cancer could become wise to the drugs and show itself. This is when the medical team would look to try me on another maintenance drug.

My parents kept hope that the Niraparib would be successful and give me what I needed to survive, but I knew they were worrying constantly about my health. They decided to book a break for us – just Mum and Dad, me, and my brother - as they felt we all needed to get away and enjoy a family holiday making more memories together. Mum and dad were on the case and had us booked to go on a cruise to Norway the following year.

In June of this year my work colleague, Chloe, in her mid-twenty's suffered a stroke. I found out what ward she was on at the hospital, and I drove there straight after work to go visit her and take some goodies to cheer her up. This, again, for my work colleagues, was another big blow they had to come to terms with. I found Chloe was more of a shock to the system than hearing my own diagnosis. She, like me, is a determined person and persisted in doing the right things to make herself well again. I kept very bubbly whilst visiting her but found my emotions inside building. You just never ever know what is waiting around that corner for you. Stories like this touch me in a big way and give me a greater appreciation of my life and those in it

As the month went on, I could feel a sensation around the area of where my ovaries used to be. Thinking about this, I had also been experiencing an aching feeling to the right side of my body, the kind of the feeling you get in your kidneys after a drinking session … not that I do that often these days! Although I feel fit and healthy, I do seem to wonder more when things like this happen as I feel so in tune with my body now since the cancer first started. Although sometimes the slightest little thing I now feel tends to put my little mind into overdrive. Not in an exaggerated state of worry but, just the fact that I always ask myself the "what if" questions. I know it's totally natural to think this way after the ordeal I have been through. I also noticed this aching happening upon waking. It could be a stitch from overdoing things, I guessed. I monitored this and noted in my journal for a few days as these aches and pains occurred. *I can let the team know at my next clinic* I thought. '*I mean, they have totally got my back', what could possibly get past me now?'*

The month continued and saw my time between filled with various appointments and time was spent well with friends and family. A trip to Copenhagen with my usual gang of misfits did me the world of good to get away from it all and just have a change of scenery, and such a great tonic for me. We all travelled to Copenhagen to visit our friend Kat who was working there at the time. Copenhagen is full of history as well as modern architecture and most of its population ride bicycles to get around the city. In fact, I have never seen so many bicycles in a city, and they take precedence over the pedestrians (literally). We always had to be careful when crossing roads, because these Danish cyclists were taking no prisoners with them! Our trip took us to many fascinating places, meeting wonderful people along the way. We did a chilled day out at the Tivoli Gardens and took a visit to the Carlsberg City, where Kat was working. I remember the brewery tour well and sampling various flavoured beers with added herbs and spices to tickle our taste buds.

At the end of June my friend, Jeni's son, Reaghan, came over from the USA to England to go on an archaeological dig up North of the map. He stayed with my family for a few days, and we took him to a few places of interest. Between my friends and family, we packed in quite a bit from pub lunches, Stonehenge, a trip to Bath – a historical city full of amazing architecture - and a pub crawl around Winchester town – another great town full of history and character.

At the end of Reaghan's stay, I drove him up to Birmingham train station to drop him off and say my goodbyes, before heading across to my friends Jac and Johnny to spend a few days with them. An emotional day for me to say goodbye and feeling the worry his mother probably felt when she said goodbye to him at Phoenix airport in the USA. Although young, in mind he is old and wise enough to look after himself, but as I said my goodbyes, turned my back and began to walk away, it didn't stop me shedding a few tears. I felt like he was kind of my responsibility and now it was out of my hands as he went onwards on his journey up country to his dig.

On the upside of this, my blood results came back with an amazing blood count of just fifteen point three. Such a great result considering eleven months ago they were up in the eight hundred figures. The activity had calmed down in my body and my bloods were going in the right direction. My parents were gobsmacked at how quickly this was all turning around for me. Time passed and I continued positively on with my life, catching up with family and friends, and getting out with my camera.

* * *

Chapter Fourteen

Tess

My friend, Jo, is another one in life who has had rubbish thrown at her over the years with ill health and operations. Jo is an amazing girl because she never grumbles, and nothing phases her. She has various health issues and yet she is gutsy, always laughing and telling dirty jokes and lives life with a smile all the way. The same goes for Jo's sister, Tess.

I met Tess, back in the summer of 2015. Tess had just finished her chemotherapy treatment and was in Southampton spending time with Jo and Matt. I had popped over a few times during her stay there to spend time chilling with a few drinks and having a bit of a laugh. This was long before I was diagnosed, and we sat talking about her experience. There came a time through Tess's ordeal, when she was told there was nothing more the surgeons and specialist could do for her. Tess was not giving up without a fight and refused to leave the consultant's room until they agreed to help her further. Eventually they told Tess there was one thing left they were willing to try for her own personal situation, and that was giving her a chemo bath operation. Tess felt she had nothing to lose, and for her, money was no object. Her life was the centre of everything, and she was prepared to do what it took to keep herself alive. She had discussed the chemo bath procedure with her consultant. It was not going to be a safe and easy operation. Tess fully understood what she was letting herself in for but in her eyes, if she didn't go through with the major operation, she "would" die, and if she took a 50/50 chance in knowing she "might" die, then there was no question about it. Tess was all in and agreed to go ahead.

It was nearing the time for Tess to undergo her own operation. I did not realise at the time how much this was scaring her because she seemed her happy, jolly self, always having a laugh and brushing it off.

Tess and I had discussed going to photograph the blood moon. This was happening the night before her operation. We decided that we would take our cameras and go to Salisbury Cathedral, in the hope of capturing some good shots. We had done our research and social media reported the moon would be visible for the night of September 27th and on into the following morning. The rare blood-red eclipse would last just over an hour, occurring in the early hours at around 3am. Yes, mad we both were but it was a special night for Tess to forget the trauma her body was about to go through.

It was late when I picked Tess up and we set off in my car to Salisbury. As we drove towards the city, we could see the tall spire in the distance. In fact, you can't miss it! The cathedral is situated right in the town centre and it has the tallest church spire in the UK at just over four-hundred feet; it is one of many stunning English architecture sites I have been fortunate to visit. We drove up to a set of large wooden gates to find that the place was closed. Well, we didn't think that one through, did we?! Inside the gates lived a small community of people in the courtyard so I guess this is closed at night for that reason. We walked around part of the perimeter to see if we could find another way to get in or climb over, but it was impossible. Twenty minutes passed and we were back in the car keeping warm and pondering what we should do. We had our flask of coffee and munchies in the car so being fed and watered was not going to be an issue. I heard a noise and looked up.

"Tess look, there's a guy coming out of the gates."

As soon as I had spoken Tess jumped out of the car and walked over to greet him. We chatted with him for a bit about our disappointment and laid it on about how we had driven "so far" to come and photograph the blood moon backdropped against the cathedral.

"Well girls, I don't actually live here. I'm looking after my friends place whilst he's away travelling."

We chatted some more with him and then he walked back to the gates, unlocked them, turned, and looked at us, and told us to drive the car in, be quiet during our stay within the cathedral grounds and to be sure when we left the premises that we shut the gates behind us. Although gobsmacked he was allowing us in, I was not turning the opportunity down, and within minutes we said our goodbyes and we were in. We felt like naughty children as we knew we shouldn't be there and that at any time anyone could walk out from their property to ask why we were there. We enjoyed the moment talking, giggling, taking photos, and strolling around the cathedral grounds and we sure made the most of our visit. The early hours drew in and we decided it was time to leave and get Tess back home. She needed to get some rest before her next ordeal was about to start.

Tess later told me that evening meant so much to her and took her mind off everything running over in her head and going on around her. She said this night out was what she needed. Something fun and positive to focus on and take her away from the world of CANCER.

Tess has undergone numerous amounts of surgery and treatments to battle cancer. She has been cut from here to Timbuktu and had so much removed. But that is her story and not for me to be writing about. I just wanted to share what a strong, positive, and special person she really is. No matter what she may have been feeling inside, Tess kept calm and carried on. How she manages to keep her zest for life, is beyond me. Tess is one incredible person and one that truly deserves a mention in my story. She has certainly inspired me on my journey.

* * *

Chapter Fifteen

Ugly

My friend's wedding was just around the corner, and I was glad I was fit and well enough to attend.

Amongst the excitement, inside I didn't feel very womanly, or myself. I stood there looking at my reflection in the mirror and I didn't like what I saw. I didn't feel beautiful or attractive or likeable or interesting. I saw someone different looking back at me. My hair was short and brown, and although I had it cut into a style to try to suit me for the day, I didn't like it and I felt somewhat butch looking. The steroids had bloated my face and my body. Steroids can change the shape of the eye lens, too, and they draw in water which makes the eyes look a lot fatter.

This was one time when I didn't feel my best and truly hated the way I looked. The more I tried to find an outfit to wear that made me feel good, the less I was finding the right thing, and I hated the shape of my body.

Wow, for such a positive person this was sure beginning to knock my confidence. I thought about how I had got stuck in the shallow aesthetics of it all. I have never judged others as I was now judging myself. So I didn't understand why now my looks seemed to be a current issue for me, making me feel so withdrawn and anxious. Maybe it was a natural post treatment feeling people get?

I contemplated several times and kept going over the same ground, yet I knew deep down that nothing was stopping me from going to the wedding of my dear friends. Just because I had issues with how I looked and felt right then it shouldn't stop me from being with those I love. For sure they would be horrified if they knew I was worrying about my looks or didn't show because of this. I just need to put on a brave face and get out there, to party with my friends and to enjoy the weekend, and so I did.

* * *

Chapter Sixteen

Relapse

I was sent a letter to attend the Princess Anne Hospital for my next clinic. That meant only one thing to me. My bloods probably were not playing ball, and I was right. The results were showing a slow incline back up to 63.4. At least I was being checked and the hospital totally had my back with it all, so hopefully, catching this activity early, would help them to help me get this sorted out again. I had a work masquerade ball to go to in the evening so at least that was another exciting event to put it to the back of my mind and go have some fun.

Christmas was spent with my parents and brother, and it was the first time we had spent several days together like this since I could remember. I wanted time to stand still, I didn't want this to end. It's the moments like this, and the memories made that you must cherish, because you never get them back again.

The rest of the Christmas holidays took me to restaurants with friends and seeing in the new year. But what was meant to be the start of a happy new year, and I was back at the main General hospital with my cousin, Sarah, to go back through all the rigmarole of my usual check-ups and CT scans.

We were then with Dr Green in her office talking things over.

"What did you say? One hundred and thirty-eight? my bloods are at one hundred and thirty-eight?" I questioned.

My heart sank as I was told this news. At that moment I was so wishing it would be something less sinister but deep down I knew this was my arch enemy paying me another visit.

"Jackie the chances of you being cured just with the chemotherapy was always slim. We would be looking to use the Niraparib anti-body treatment when it becomes available to us. This is looking likely to be around the time we expect your treatment to finish, which is quite promising".

I didn't get it; I was feeling good that day. Yeah, I suffered with pangs to my left side, but I was generally okay in myself. I thought I was reading my body well, and I put the pangs down to the possibility that the chemo was killing off the cancer cells, so cancer was not at the forefront of my mind. I genuinely thought there would be nothing to worry about.

Dr Green continued, "the nodule in your peritoneum cavity is at 6mm. There is also scar tissue there which is what is causing your intermittent pangs. The scars can snag the bowel occasionally." My cousin was constantly writing and asking questions for me as she could see from my face that the cogs were ticking over inside. Sarah asked questions that I had not thought of or just forgot because I was listening to what was being explained to me and still had that number echoing in my head one, three, eight. There is always so much information to take in and talk about, and it can become tiring at times. We left the hospital arm in arm to go have a stiff drink.

Amongst the doom and gloom, I carried on with being focused, and by the first week of February I was north of the map in Liverpool. I met up with a small group of photographers to learn about long exposure photography. This event was organised by Matt Hart. I have followed Matt for a few years, and he is known for his love of Fuji cameras and street photography. Matt is good at bringing together a wide skillset of people within the photography community to travel to cities and mountainous regions across the country to have fun whilst taking photographs. He himself, has had his health issues to overcome, yet he always encourages others to get out there, see the world, enjoy the moment, and capture it with pictures. Due to Matt and his team, I have met so many wonderful characters and it has helped me gain back some of the confidence I lost when I was too sick to get out using my camera for months.

Many who attend these photography days have their own trials and tribulations and things like this give us a purpose and gets us out of our comfort zones. When doing something new or meeting new people, it has my heart racing with excitement teamed with complete fear and anxiety. Living on my own means I have no one to answer to, so if I did not push myself to do such things for enjoyment, I wouldn't do anything or meet anyone. Photography is my passion and having this hobby has been a huge help to me. I also love to share my work with the world. Anyone reading this who knows me will agree I take a lot of pictures! Whether it be on my travels, walking with nature, street photography, etc - this is when I am most content. I am no David Bailey, but when I make people smile with my pictures, then that makes me happy.

After a good day out, I left the group and drove my way down to Bromsgrove to be with Jacquie and Johnny and lay my hat for the night. For Jac and I, it was feet up whilst giving our arms a good workout lifting our wine glasses, as our lovely Johnny put his culinary skills into action. The whole weekend distracted my mind for a bit, yet I still knew I had a bit of a trek to go on the medical side of things.

Over the next couple of weeks my tummy was feeling irritated. I had a show of back passage bleeding. One minute I had a constipated feeling and the next I was rushing to get to the toilet in time. I began to worry there might be large tumours pressing heavily inside again. I was not liking my body shape. I have never had a large stomach, so this was a marker for me, a confirmation in my mind that the cancer was back. I continued eating a low fibre diet to prevent gas and raised my water intake to help with the dehydration. I had refluxes starting to occur, so I ensured I had plenty of Movicol sachets to try to resolve this quickly before my cruise in May. I began to purchase the next size up in clothing so I would have a comfier choice to consider nearing the holiday. All I could do was continue to do things to help myself, continue as my medical team advised and keep living with hope.

I was in and out of hospital for bloods and signing BRCA testing consent forms to help the hospital with further investigations. Because my bloods were now up to 934, they needed to be sure of where the cancer may have spread to and so I was sent for more scans to check my upper chest area.

"Your chest scan results are really good, Jackie, and not showing any signs of cancer spread; however, there is something microscopic which has been very slowly growing over the past few months and it looks like you have a tumour on your spleen of about 20mm. This won't go away and will always be there."

We sat talking through my questions. The next step was to have my bloods tested to see if I had mutations within the tumour. If this was so, then it would give me a better chance to have the Niraparib drug and for us to work towards maintaining the cancer that has chosen to squat in my spleen against my wishes.

My bloods were due to be taken on my first cycle of my second lot of chemotherapy sessions.

Many people ask me why the surgeons cannot just take away my spleen as it is not a vital organ, and one I can live without. I had asked my consultant, Dr Green, that very same question. To try to explain this in a nutshell, the cancer is a bit like blowing a dandelion. The little seedlings scatter within your body. When these find somewhere to attach, they then start to grow and spread. Due to the BRCA testing, and the fact the cancer is currently mutating within the tumour, it is safer for me to maintain this and keep it at bay, rather than remove my spleen and the tiny, microscopic cancer seedlings finding somewhere else, such as a vital organ to attach itself to.

I have found some of the information I have researched to be very confusing at times, and I still must go back and read up on certain things now to get a better understanding. I think I sometimes tie myself up in knots with the many questions I continue to pose to doctors, and I ask repeated questions at my clinics. Dr Green and her team have always been fine with my inquisitions. That is what they are there for, to help and guide their patients with their knowledge and support and to keep going over old ground with anything you do not fully understand. I think

I was either a breath of fresh air to them or a complete pain in the ass.

Without delving into the wonderful world of science too much, I wanted to touch on the maintenance drugs I am now taking daily for life.

Niraparib (Zejula) or Bevacizumab (Avastin) are PARP inhibitors and are prescribed as a maintenance treatment for adult patients with recurrent epithelial ovarian, fallopian tube, or primary peritoneal cancer, who are in a complete or partial response to platinum-based chemotherapy, such as Carboplatin.

To grow, the cancer needs a good blood supply. Once the tumour has grown to around the size of 2mm, it then needs to grow its own blood vessels to be able to continue to grow.

Some cancers make a protein which attaches to cell receptors. These receptors line the walls of blood vessels within the malignant tumour and cause the blood vessels to grow, resulting in the cancer being able to grow.

Niraparib is a "holding measure" and plays an important role by interfering with the growth of new blood vessels to the malignant tumour and stopping the protein from helping damaged cells repair themselves.

PARP inhibiters can stop the repair process from happening in damaged ovarian cancer cells which causes the cells to weaken and die.

"Jackie, the hospital will send off your bloods to the Salisbury Genetics Lab and the results take four to six weeks to come back. However, I am incredibly happy with how your bloods are responding and you will be given the Niraparib drug independent of the BRCA result. We do need to get you started on the Niraparib. Apart from the spleen, everything is lying dormant. Your cancer is not curable, but we can supress it with Niraparib. These drugs are the parp inhibitors we previously discussed, which will help to keep the cancer maintained for a while. You may experience some side effects with this, the most common are insomnia and nausea, which is short lived. I suggest you pick a regular time to take these, and you must keep within that time window as much as possible."

Wow, I thought, *what a great combination of side effects that is*. If I were to take the drugs in the morning/day, I would be wide awake but feel sick, and if I took the drugs in the evening, I could take them before bed and that would combat the nausea feeling as I would be asleep however, this then counteracts with experiencing the insomnia. *What is the point of that?* I thought about this, and I decided to go with the latter of the two and I would start taking the drugs at ten o'clock every night before bed.

I wanted to know how long this was going to keep the disease at bay. Dr Green couldn't tell me, which is understandable. She explained that she was gauging this on the effects of past maintenance drugs on patients using Niraparib, and at a guess she thought these would buy me about 5 or 6 months. I mean, how long is a piece of string, right? It isn't something you can always put a time limit on, and I guess in a good way, I'm better off just getting on with the fight and living a happy healthy life, rather than thinking about how many months, days, weeks, hours, or minutes I might have left to live.

The plan was to give me the Carbo Platin and Gemcitabine of 4 to 6 cycles, then start me on the Niraparib drug once it becomes available to the NHS. It's all down to the timing of the research, trials, and funding as to when such drugs can be made available to the hospitals. I prayed the sooner the better as I wanted them to be ready and prescribed to me once my treatment ended. I didn't want another waiting game on my hands at this stage.

Luckily, this was something where the hospital could fit my treatment plan around me. There would be no loss of hair with the second lot of chemotherapy treatment. It would not be as harsh as before and a much kinder treatment to me.

The cycles would be approximately two hours once set up, so at least I wouldn't have to pack for England when I went to the sessions. As before I would have a lower immune system (neutropenia) the second week after each chemo cycle.

Dr Green told me I would have blood tests every week for a month after treatment and then monthly thereafter, to keep a close check on how I was doing. If the platelets showed as being low then the hospital would look to drop my dosage of the Niraparib, to allow my white blood cells time to recover.

I began to ask more questions … as if the medical team had not heard enough questions from me already!

"Can you tell me if the cancer has gone to any lymph nodes in that area?"

"No, it hasn't. The cancer has grown quickly and is a high-grade type 3."

"If this is the case, then why are fewer toxic drugs being administered to me this time?"

"Due to what you have already gone through, it might be detrimental for you to have a harsher dosage of these drugs to combat this."

"I know this sounds like a stupid question; however, you say that the CA125 blood tests show high levels of protein. Should I lessen the amount of protein I eat?"

"Firstly, do not feel any question you ask is a silly one, Jackie." Dr Green looked at me and smiled, "please always ask away no matter how trivial you feel it might be, that is what we are here for. The answer to your question is no, Jackie, eating food containing protein has nothing to do with why you have high levels of protein in your blood. This is completely different and the protein we talk about in your blood is tumour related."

Dr Green always welcomed my many questions, and although I had an appointment time slot, she had time for me, as she did with everyone walking through that door. Our conversations never felt rushed and as though it was a one in, one out scenario and I always came away feeling that I'd been listened to and with knowledge gained that I understood well.

Once I relapsed, I honestly believed my cancer had returned with a vengeance due to what I had been feeding my body, and although natural sugars, it was still a large sugar consumption overall. I was too focused on blitzing lots of fruits together rather than the right fruits and balancing them out in my diet

* * *

Chapter Seventeen

Sugar Coated

I continued to research further into low sugar and what I was putting into my body. I was understanding a little more about the science behind food, and this was another minefield, believe me! Although this seemed like a huge task, I kept to reading bite size chunks of information so as not to cloud my mind.

Most of us are knowledgeable with regards to eating healthy, and foods that can be bad for you. From past knowledge and what I began to understand from my research, enzymes in foods can break down differently when cooked or processed in some way; for example, blending fruits does not benefit your body as much as eating them whole. You lose the goodness because of the processing and what you are blitzing together. If you think about it, it is the same principle as not boiling your vegetables into oblivion as you are just boiling out the goodness into the water, which is why it is better to lightly steam vegetables or eat them raw to retain the nutritional goodness.

You should of course never prep meat and vegetables on the same chopping board due to harmful bacteria that breed and could make you sick. Being a cancer patient, things like this are paramount when trying to keep your body healthy and fit for battle!

I started to believe that by blending a large variety of fruits together and drinking them throughout the day, I was probably actually doing more harm than good. If you are going to process food in some way then the best way to ensure you are putting the right ingredients together is to research online, purchase healthy eating or anti-cancer recipe books, and get advice from the charity centres because some of them do keep recipe books for cancer patients. Talking to family and friends about this is helpful. It will only make life easier for you if you can also get your loved ones on board, so they understand you are being serious about your health. There is so much information now on social media as well as books, and I choose my internet browsing wisely. I tend to stick to a few good books and google the science when I need to know more.

One evening whilst visiting my friends Lynne and Steve, we began discussing my illness and the kinds of things I was doing to try to help my body get as much goodness as possible. I explained about the amount of sugar I was packing into my body daily with smoothies and various other foods, and how I felt it could be feeding my cancer rather than starving it.

I mentioned to Lynne that I felt as though I was feeding my body with too much sugar from blending many kinds of fruits together because of the brief research I'd done on the subject. I was starting to believe that sugar was feeding my cancer, hence why I relapsed, and I personally believed this was why the cancer returned so quickly. I expressed my feelings for wanting to cut as much sugar out of my diet as possible to see if this would make a difference.

Lynne asked me to try something sweet she had made and put in the freezer. She took out what looked like broken pieces of Dime bars and allowed them to slightly defrost. It was an after-dinner dessert consisting of cocoa, raspberries, and coconut oil. Lynne makes this low sugar treat to eat and stop her cravings for too many sugary based things. It tasted different and the coconut oil made the texture feel slick as it melted in my mouth and ran down the back of my throat, but I liked it.

"Jackie, I'm going to show you this book that I've been using." Lynne left the kitchen and came back with book in hand. I did this last year for a health kick and then I stopped. Recently I've started to feel sluggish and bloated, so I began using this book again."

The book was called I Quit Sugar by a lady called Sarah Wilson. It's a low sugar cookbook. Lynne said once she started, she lived religiously by the low sugar eating and stuck to the menu choices from the recipe book. She explained that by doing this, it became quite noticeable that she was losing the extra weight because she was sticking to the food plans and had cut out alcohol.

I was looking to find a diet not for weight loss reasons but to feed my body with what it needed, and this book sounded perfect for what I wanted to achieve.

As Lynne continued to talk about the recipes, I picked up the book and flicked through the pages. Straight away I liked the layout of the book. It wasn't too brain taxing and very easy to follow. I could choose to read it step by step or dip in and out of the pages to find which low sugar recipes I fancied making. This was a definite need for my bookshelf, and I thought if I could start by introducing low sugar food most of the time, then this would be a step in the right direction in helping my body to digest and retain the nutrients better in my system.

"Jackie, some things might taste a bit different to start with, especially if you are a person who has a sweet tooth, or you like very rich foods but if you can get past those barriers, it's worth trying."

I love this book for its variety of low sugar recipes, which include cakes and desserts you can incorporate into your meal plans. Sarah, the author, is Australian. She's a health coach and journalist, and what started out for her as a kind of new year's resolution experiment, has now stuck and she is several healthy eating books in.

I wanted a diet I could believe in, something good to feed me to good health, something to maybe starve or prevent my cancer spreading. I wanted to ensure that what I put into my body was the right food, and food to make me feel good inside and out.

Mobile phone out - internet on – Amazon – ordered - Bam! … job done!

Its arrival that week in the post excited me. I started by trying just 3 recipes in the first couple of weeks, then as I continued to read on through the book, I introduced the next two or three recipes and so on.

I love this book because it doesn't bombard you with too much food science. Sarah Wilson touches on the science side of things but, explains in the book that if you wish to know more, to google it. I feel this stops a lot of confusion compared to some books that go heavy on the science side of things. It's an easy-to-understand book that walks you through the stages so that you can take what you want from it and experiment a bit at a time to get the most from it, rather than becoming too overwhelmed with the information or getting bored of reading too much text before getting to the recipe sections.

My favourite to date is the sausage and beetroot breakfast hash. Some recipe ingredients might sound a little weird, but I think most work, and it is about just trying new things and maybe adjusting your taste buds a bit.

My small bit of research had made me think about what I was putting into my body, and I personally feel that too much sugar feeds cancer so I needed to do what I could to starve the cancer from what it was craving. Cancer cells cannot be starved alone by cutting out sugar, but I feel by fuelling my body and my skin with goodness, and keeping it nourished, along with taking the Niraparib, I am helping to deflect the illness as much as possible so I will live longer.

I started by making small changes and swapping things out or finding low sugar alternatives. My energy levels began to rise, and my skin started to look clearer. If the changes I'd made to my diet were doing this to my external appearance, I could only imagine the good it must be doing to my internal organs. I feel that by persevering enough, you will notice small differences over time, and it becomes easier.

I eat twice as healthy as before and make wiser food choices. When I shop, I do check food labels for the 'Carbohydrates of which sugars.' I try to stick to a rule of under 5g per item, and the lower the better. At the beginning this was hard work as the same foods manufactured as different brands had a completely different sugar content, so checking the labels started out to be very time consuming. Now I do this regularly and it's has become less of a chore, and it interests me to see what unexpected items contain a large amount of sugar. Things such as low-fat yoghurt or granola seem like a healthy option, and yet they have a high sugar content. I use plant-based milk in my drinks now, and I have changed to decaffeinated tea and coffee, and I have green tea with a slice of lemon and root ginger.

Some people get confused and believe eating low fat foods is healthier for you than full fat items. This is sometimes down to how they are marketed, normally with a healthy, fit looking person holding the low fat (full of sugar) product on a TV advertisement.

Don't think that low sugar products fall into the same category as low fat = THEY DO NOT. Most products advertise their goods as being low in fat but generally hold a lot of sugar or synthetic sugary tasting substitutes.

I have noticed in some conversations I have about my diet, that some people instantly recommend or talk to me about low fat foods. They seem to think my new diet consists of me eating a lot of products that state they are low in fat - I do NOT! I eat full fat, which is lower in sugar.

When I decided to start the diet, I emptied my cupboards of all stock items containing over five grams of sugar. Well, that was most of my food gone! I now make my own coconutty granola (thank you Sarah Wilson), sauces, salad dressings and regularly cook world cuisine rather than eating too many takeaways, but! … I will give myself the occasional takeaway as a treat. The more I know what is going in my food, the better I feel I can help my body to control the cancer and retain the right nutrients. I eat less red meat now as this can be a big help on the bowels and digestive system. It is all about gaining extra knowledge, learning to say no and being more in control of your food choices

We are always taught through life to "eat up our greens" and "an apple a day keeps the doctor away". These things I talk of are not new to us and it has all been said time and time before. I just want to highlight to people going through cancer, that even though I have generally eaten a good diet, I have made significant changes that I believe have helped prolong my life and could save it in the long run.

My cancer is not curable and since I have been on this diet, and taking my maintenance drugs, the cancer has been lying dormant in my spleen. My skin and hair feel better, I feel more energetic, and I don't experience as much nausea on the drugs as I first did, so that can only be a good sign.

I thought back to my first ovarian cancer diagnosis with my red blood cells up in the eight hundreds. And then to get a secondary cancer diagnosis for my spleen, with bloods which had metastasised to the thousands. I believe there were microscopic seedlings left behind after the first lot of treatments and operation, and by way of my diet at that time, I was keeping the seedlings alive, and they resided on my spleen. Even though this still could have come back, if I had been doing the low sugar diet from the very start, then just maybe they may not have returned so aggressively, or just maybe I could have done my part in killing it off and keeping it away?

This was what spiralled me into my researching frenzy to gain knowledge on how I could help myself. Therefore, I chose to eat a diet low in sugar and stop blitzing lots of fruit together, as I personally felt, although fruit sugars are better than refined sugars, I was giving my body a sugar overload, and feeding the cancer on what it needed to survive. Some foods are healthier when eaten on their own rather than after they have been processed in some way. It is just a case of knowing what you are doing, when purchasing and prepping your food. I don't always get it right but at least I am trying and sticking to my beliefs. My smoothies now consisted mainly of vegetables or only blending the fruits recommended from my anti-cancer smoothie book. I would only add one fruit to the vegetable smoothies such as an apple or a pear to sweeten it, but the rest of the smoothie consisted of veg and looked like something a frog would swim in. If I wanted more fruit in my diet, I mainly ate it unprepared.

The one thing sticking in my mind was keeping my body healthy and keeping me alive for longer. I didn't mind drinking these smoothies and I added things like turmeric that would benefit my recovery due to their anti-inflammatory and antioxidant properties. I treat my body even better than I already did before and show it more love now that it has been through the battlefield. An illness can age your body and therefore, if you can do good leading up to, during and after treatment, then this will help you with your recovery process and living as normal a life as possible.

I often spoke of this when at my hospital clinics, yet the hospital seemed reluctant to confirm anything as being good or bad. What might work for me might not work for another.

A good place to start is by introducing small changes (even if just cutting down on your refined sugar intake), making more healthy choices, researching various alternatives, and preparing food correctly. 'I Quit Sugar' teaches you just that in an easy eight-week plan to get you going with easy-to-follow snippets throughout the book. You can dip in and out of and most of the ingredients you need to purchase are used throughout the book in various recipes and there are good tips on using up leftovers from other meals.

Healthy eating reduces the risk of bowel cancer, helps with weight loss and therefore, reducing obesity which can also reduce the risk of cancer.

Many of the cancer charities have good recipes to follow on their websites or on leaflets at their centres. Not all these will be actual low sugar cookbooks, but they will include healthy easy to follow recipes. You can contact the centres or pop in to pick up a copy.

I think for someone with any illness, by finding foods and drinks that are good in building a healthy body up, and retain nutrients within the body, only helps the body from doing too much hard work itself with breaking down the enzymes; and by cutting out as many of the bad things as you can, it will do good in helping your body to repair itself and keep the cancer at bay/rid yourself of it completely

Chapter Eighteen

Cruising the Calm before Stormy Seas

Saturday May 19th, 2018, and we were ready to embark on our long-awaited adventure on our Norwegian Cruise. For someone who was not at all fussed about doing a cruise, it proved to be everything and more. From boarding and being able to start our holiday straight away, to fine dining and dressing up for the Captain's Dinner, it felt good to be away together. The only downfall was spending my first full day sick on board the Azura ship whilst docked at Stavanger. I could not get out of bed and lay there nursing a cold and feeling nauseous, so the best thing for me to do was just sleep. Our second day we docked at Flam. I felt better and made the effort to get myself up and take a shower. Just the feeling of the warm running water trickling over the top of my head and down over my body gave me a feel-good factor straight away. I just stood there for a moment, eyes closed, mindful of the sensation and temperature of the water and just trying to block out negativity and how my body was struggling.

Once I was ready, next on the agenda was a nice, cooked breakfast from the buffet. I was looking forward to getting out to see the beauty of the Fjords and making my use of the ship's fine dining, eating, and drinking our way through the restaurants and the buffets. Well, I had to make the bloody most of this trip as it was not going to be plain sailing upon our return.

Our parents took the early train trip up to the mountains. My brother and I took the later one as we wanted to do a bike ride back down the mountains. The train took us up and then halfway back down it stopped, and we got off at a little platform with a few others who had also booked bicycle hire. We took a ride down the rest of the way - luckily for me it was all downhill, so I knew this would be a breeze for me. En route we occasionally stopped to take in the stunning picturesque snow-capped mountains, the warmth of the sunshine and flowing waterfalls bellowing down the sides and tops of the mountains. May time was the best time for us to go, as the spring brings everything to life and as the snow begins to melt, so the waterfalls begin to appear in their cascading glory. Such a breath -taking experience which gave me a sense of calm and inner peace and will live in my memory forever. I remember breathing in the clean fresh air with an earthy pine scent. It was so fresh and crisp, and my mind was beginning to empty. I felt free from thinking too hard, free from asking lists of questions, free from being jabbed with needles and cannulas, free from my cancer life for just a while. I felt happy, I felt alive, and I felt like a piece of me again.

The evenings were a different story, and they took their toll on me. Every time after dinner we would chill in the piano bar or go see a show followed by a night cap, well for me anyway. My evenings always ended with me starting to flag and one of my family walking me back to my cabin early to go to bed. The three of them would then carry on the night together. Later, back home in England, we were talking about the holiday one evening, and discussing how tired I had been in the evenings, and then about Tony sitting alone on deck watching the beautiful Norwegian sunsets until gone 11 o'clock at night. This inwardly upset me and made me feel emotional that the one amazing experience we all had together, and I felt too tired in my body to stay up and share these wonderful moments with my brother. He always says he did not mind, but I sometimes wonder what thoughts he had in his alone time on that ship.

Ten days passed from when we first boarded the Azura and what seemed like yesterday to me was now in the distance, and I was back in hospital for more clinics, more tests, and form filling to give my consent for more chemo treatment, for the next lot of shrinkage and post control of my tumours with the maintenance drugs. These tumours were resting on my rectum and stomach lining, and there was still the 23mm tumour on my spleen.

I was asked to follow a low fibre fact sheet for the first 2 cycles to help with my bowel movements. Thereafter a high fibre diet could commence again. As before: week one I would have nausea and tiredness, week two: the constipation and risk of infection and week three would be a normal week, although I wasn't sure what normal was anymore.

I kept faith with all the circus going on around me and still socialising with people when I could, whilst sticking to as much low sugar foods as possible. I felt more in control, and if my beliefs meant choosing alternatives or missing out much of the time to keep sugar from feeding my cancer, then that was what I would do. Yes, I had my naughty days, but I stuck to being as healthy as possible to build up my immune system to combat the fact that my bone marrow was not working quickly enough to do this for me.

I took counselling sessions at Jane Scarth House, had my monthly clinics, and endured more chemo treatments. I had a few bouts of sickly days, but I kept thinking about the fact that this poison travelling around inside me was what was killing off the cancer cells to get me well again.

My next clinic was on June 21st at the Princess Anne, for my blood results. This unnerved me as I normally got told bad news when asked to attend this building rather than the General Hospital across the road. My appointment was with Dr Akis, one of Dr. Green's team. Dr Akis welcomed me and my parents in and we talked of how I had been reacting to treatment and how I was feeling. I just wanted the niceties done and for him to give me the lowdown on things. Dr Akis got to the vital part, and he confirmed my bloods were remarkable. I paused for a moment and then when I questioned this, he told me my blood cells were showing as being normal in shape and size, and that he was happy by this change.

It was not until I was back home from my appointment, and still chewing this over, that it then dawned on me just maybe my food changes could be helping to contribute to my bloods starting to look normal. I continued as I was going and took more counselling and Reiki sessions at Jane Scarth between my hospital treatments and appointments to help me keep relaxed and stress free.

July 6th, I went to see Roger Walters from Pink Floyd play in London's Hyde Park with my friends. Before the gig I met up with Missy, another friend from America. It was a scorching hot day and after I left Missy, I made my way into the gates to go wait inside the entrance for my friends. I took a slow walk around the event to see what other activities were taking place pre-event, and then I waited for a couple of hours for my friends to turn up. They had stopped off to have a few drinks en route and waiting seemed like forever to me. The heat was too hot to handle and at one point I started feeling queasy and thought I might pass out. I found a tree with a bit of shade but everyone else had the same idea, and it ended up with people cramming into the shaded areas to try to keep cool. I was getting restless and moved back into the sunshine. I felt too shy to play the cancer card and ask for people to move for me so I could keep cool. Just as I thought I could not take much more, my friend texted to say they were not far from the park. I kept well hydrated drinking as much water as I could, and once they arrived, I felt the anxiety fading away and the calm making an entrance. We pitched up a spot on the grass facing the stage and waited for the music to take a hold of us. I never told my friends how I really felt that day or how scared I was feeling, but my spirits lifted once I knew I wasn't alone, and we all enjoyed a great evening together singing Pink Floyd songs as the sun was setting.

As the days passed, I thought more about everything, and my main worry was that if I left my family behind, how would they deal with it? I think sometimes it was too much for them to take on board when we went to see my consultant. We'd go in and then I would always forget things I should have asked because my mind was on how my parents were feeling. Also, I felt there were things I needed to discuss with the consultant that they did not need to hear about; things that were personal to me, so I found this difficult discussing how I was feeling or what my body was doing, when we were all sat there in the room together.

It was a stressful time and although your loved ones will want to be there and do everything for you, if you feel you need space or want to go to an appointment on your own then you need to tell them so.

I learned that I needed to start going to certain appointments on my own so that I could have my own time with the consultant instead of worrying about what my parents would have to listen to.

It might sound selfish of me, however, this had to be about me and my needs, I was the one going through this, no one else. I knew all my loved ones wanted to protect and support me but there were times when I felt the need to have time alone with my consultant so that I could ask my questions fully take in what I was being told.

Some may not understand this as they may always want to have another person there by their side. I'm grateful for all the love and support I've had, and the strong and positive attitude of those around me; however, as far as I was concerned this was a good lesson learned for me, and God forbid this should happen again, then at least I know I can deal with it and attend certain appointments on my own when I need to.

From August right through to November time I suffered with the aching bones, uncomfortable pains, the visits back and forth to clinics for CT scans, then more chemo cycles, of which one was deferred due to my white blood cell count not rising quickly enough to fight infection. I had sick days off work to recoup and build my energy levels back up, then the repetitive cycle of it all again.

It seemed never ending, but I kept believing and went with the plan, listened to what I needed to do and where I needed to be and when. Time passed and my red blood count was starting to show a "nearly normal" count at long last. They had reduced right down from three hundred and forty-two point two, to forty-eight point five. I was getting closer to the goal, and I knew if we could just push this back under thirty-five then I would have conquered again.

There were more complications with a low white blood count. My

162

treatment was to be deferred further and my body was now back in the recovery stage between treatment cycles. The medical team told me the bone marrow was still not producing enough white blood cells to fight infection. The white cell count needed to be much higher and yet my CA125 red bloods were dropping nicely in the right direction. The team had to consider my safety, and so decided to compensate with a smaller dose of chemotherapy in the hope it would enable my white cell count to rise a little.

Then I had some uplifting news. Later tests results showed the drugs were doing what they said on the tin! The original tumour size of 20mm had shrunk. It went down to ten millimetres and then decreased to six millimetres.

"I have some great news, Jackie; your CA125 bloods are at two point five which is exceptionally low." Dr Green smiled. "I have never, in this hospital seen anyone with bloods to drop this low. These results are amazing, Jackie, and you've done incredibly well in how you have dealt with all this. Your positivity and determination to change your lifestyle in what you believe to be helping you, well ..." she sat back in her chair, "all I can say is to keep doing what you're doing".

Wow! I thought of various things that I had undergone to get me to this point of hearing what I needed to hear. I was astounded and yes, I do believe the effort I have put into researching what I was putting into my body was one of the most key things in all this. This, along with trying to stay stress free, making small goals to aim for, trying to live as normal a life as I could, surrounding myself with positive people, having the willpower to not be defeated, and just everything I had strived to do was now paying off. I can't do much about the cancer in my spleen. It will be there for life but if we keep going with the maintenance drugs and my good diet then surely this is the best step forwards.

Doctor Green was beaming with pride at the results on the screen and then back at me.

"Normally for someone with ovarian cancer, a six or seven is how low the red count normally decreases for patients. Only once before have I ever seen a blood count go as low as three, but never as low as this, Jackie. The cancer has shrunk right down, and I am so pleased to give you this news."

"We'll give you a break to give your bone marrow enough time to recover so we'll see you back here in January."

We said our goodbyes, had hugs and wished each other a good Christmas and I left the oncology ward with great contentment and a feeling of wanting to scream with joy. What a buzz, and what a great lead up to the Christmas period for me.

January 8th, 2019, I attended hospital to speak further about my new drug and give my consent to get my first month's supply.

We discussed the Niraparib giving me approximately another six months. Both weird and scary to know I am buying more time on my life, but I will try anything to live. The Niraparib, as I have explained is good at denying the tumour the ability to grow back and repair its DNA. My chemotherapy treatments have smashed the tumour DNA repair and now we maintain it with Niraparib drugs.

Because of what Tess had been through, I wanted to broach other avenues with Dr Green. We discussed the chemo bath, which Dr Green and her team had never heard of. We talked of the use of cannabis oil and alternative drugs to Niraparib, getting treatments abroad that could help cure me and more operations. For me the list was endless, and it was because of those who have already been in this nightmare who have spurred me on, to want to know more, to think outside the box of anything that could keep me here that little bit longer.

Dr Green again confirmed that this cancer is not curable, and we will have spates of time, on and off chemo, and putting me on different maintenance drugs, as there are other options on the market coming out all the time. She told me that the possible behaviour of this cancer is likely to scatter and spread within my body. When? We don't know. I could go on for years, or not. Life is a ticking clock for us all and I don't want to waste what time I do have.

During all my rubbish going on in the lead up to Christmas, my auntie Doris became extremely sick. Both she and my uncle Roy have had their fair share of health issues over the years, yet they are two people in life who spurred me on with their continued laughter and love. Never did I hear them moan or groan. They both just got on with life and they laughed often. My aunties and uncles play a big part in my zest for life.

Sadly, we got the news, and we lost my auntie Doris on Christmas Eve. What was meant to be a time for celebration, was a devastating loss. My childhood memories are always happy ones and as we have all grown older, I still feel like a big piece of me has been taken away when we have loss in our family. It hurts me so much, but I hold on to the good times, the laughter, and the love we all share, which helps me through my own struggles.

The New Year saw the funeral of my auntie and a lot of hospital visits. My head was all over the show as it had been a tough Christmas for our family, and I was worrying more about my uncle Roy. He has always been known to me as my Superman and I his Wonder Woman. With all that he had suffered with the loss of the love of his life, he still wanted to know how I was and that I was okay and always put my feelings before his. My family never cease to amaze me and are the most selfless and caring people I know.

Right up until March I continued to have monthly blood checks and another X-Ray was done. All was looking good.

I continued to keep focused with my photography and in April I had three pieces of my work entered in the Hampshire Photography Exhibition that was showcasing in a local shopping centre. I had been in three photography exhibitions prior to this over the years, and I felt proud to be a part of this for good reason. All monies raised that weekend were in aid of a health care charity called Naomi House and Jacksplace. This is a hospice which focuses on palliative care for terminally ill young people. Being involved in photography exhibitions for charities is my way of giving something back to help others in great need. I feel my purpose in life is just that, and I have great need to share my knowledge and experiences to others going through cancer or those trying to support their loved ones with cancer.

* * *

Chapter Nineteen

Party On

50 years old … how the bloody hell did that happen? I got here and in one piece. How, is beyond me as this is something which I never thought possible at the beginning of my ordeal. I have managed to reach half a century, a big milestone, my fiftieth birthday. I guess it is time to party on with my nearest and dearest.

The first of the celebrations started with a weekend away with the girls. I finished work on Thursday, April 25th, and I made my way down to Bournemouth to be with my friends for the evening, which was to be a chilled one before the big 50 festivities commenced. I had no idea as to where the girls were going to be taking me for the weekend or what ideas they had up their sleeves this time. I stipulated in the weeks leading up to this event that being that much older, I didn't want a repeat of my 40th celebrations and didn't want there to be a single willy in sight! Back then the girls surprised me with anything and everything they could get their hands on from penis pasta to jumping willies. The list was endless.

I really didn't think I would be here now saying these three words "MY FIFTIETH BIRTHDAY" after hearing those initial three words "IT IS CANCER". However brave and courageous I had been throughout this process, there was a tiny minuscule part of me that thought that I wouldn't make it and I would have a slow deterioration that would see me six feet under.

Upon arrival I took my things to my room then Fi and I sat drinking and chatting whilst Andy "our host with the most" cooked for us. We didn't make it a late evening as there was a lot for Fi to get done the next morning before the big weekend.

The following morning, we had breakfast and Fi and Andy got her car loaded and away she drove without me to go meet the rest of the girls at the secret destination. The plan was that Andy would drop me off later that day to give the girls time to prep.

Once it was time for Andy to get the birthday girl en route, the excitement started to kick in. Eventually we arrived at my weekend destination in Somerset after driving around a few rural countryside lanes, we pulled up into a driveway outside a little cottage.

O M G!

As soon as we parked outside the cottage, I saw large festival flags and decorations and I knew the girls had planned my own festival.

There they all stood awaiting my arrival and I could see the various décor and lights around the garden and alongside the cottage, on the door and in the windows. There was also a large annex on the side of the cottage, which was all set up for some game playing, a wine tasting event and much more fun and frolics.

The girls were right in the festival spirit right down to the fact that they had Jackfest wrist bands made. They found it amusing to act as security at the door and frisked me before putting my wrist band on and allowing me to enter the cottage for my JackFest weekend. We did a tour of our weekend residence, room by room.

They totally got me this time. I walked into a cottage filled with music and memories. We had festival posters, laminated weekend plans on lanyards, candles and lights throughout the cottage, copious amounts of alcohol and a large variety of food to keep us going. Throughout the cottage in every room, the girls placed lights and, photos of my past, along with cardboard cut outs of Johnny Depp and Keanu Reeves, plus many other surprises

The JackFest weekend consisted of many belly laughs, games, walks, pubs, photography … the list went on. Low sugar meals were prepped and cooked for me, and Karen made me a low sugar Foo Fighters birthday cake. It was in the shape of a drum kit that had the band's logo on it, and concealed inside was a small speaker playing a Foo Fighters rendition of Happy Birthday from the cake. This is one birthday I would never forget. My girls went above and beyond in what was probably the best festival I have ever been to.

A week later saw us at the Holiday Inn Hotel in Southampton. My birthday fell on May 8th; however, the weekend fell on Star Wars Day so it was inevitable I would hold my birthday on May 4th My parents wanted to treat me to this party for obvious reasons, so I could celebrate with all my loved ones. None of us knew what cards I could get dealt in the future, no one in life does, so, I wanted to party the night away, enjoy the company of everyone and make another great memory with those who mean so much to me.

My friends and I drove to town to meet my parents and brother at the venue. The party theme was USA, and I ordered and made a lot of my own décor as well as using most of the cardboard cut outs and bunting the girls had decorated the cottage with. The DJ arrived and we spent the afternoon listening to some tunes whilst getting the place decorated in true Hollywood style.

Music plays a big part in our lives. It is with us through the good times, it with us through the bad, it reminds us of people, places, and situations. Throughout my treatment I played a wide variety of music to get me through it and keep up my spirits. I grew up listening to a lot of eighties rock and pop music and there will always be certain "stand out" songs that bring back memories of a time in your life or will have a personal meaning to you. During the period of going through my cancer, I heard a couple of songs by singers John Newman and Sean Mendez.

John Newman made a big comeback from a long-term illness with his song called Fire in Me. This is a powerful song which strongly resonates with me, as does Sean Mendez hit In My Blood.

In My Blood was not a song from one of my long-time favourite musicians. It just suddenly appeared, playing on the radio around that time, and straight away I knew this was the song! Tess called it my fight song, but I like to think of it as my comeback song, and it was the song I wanted playing at my party. It was the one I had playing in the background whilst I gave my speech. The words in that song probably mean something different to Sean Mendez, but I took from it what I wanted it to mean to me and my experience. And yes, I got to say "May the 4th be with you" at the end of my thank you speech. I was damn sure to squeeze that Star Wars line in one way or another.

The 8th and 10th saw in both mine and my dad's birthdays, and then by the 18th May my family and friends met at a local park for a Mad Hatters Tea Party picnic. Obviously, the theme was hats and we all brought along blankets, bunting, food, and drink. We had games for the kids to play on the field, and the sun was shining down on us. I couldn't have asked for more. My birthday celebrations had been well exhausted and after all this, made me quite exhausted, too!

Cancer was not going to get the better of me. Many things such as my diet have contributed to getting me here today to tell it my way.

This book highlights some of the many challenges I have had to face. I stood up to cancer and faced it head on and I pray this book will give hope to someone else going through this, or affected by this, or any other illness.

It is easy to tell someone to be brave or it will be alright, and I want you to know that whether you have a large support network or not, there is help out there in all shapes and forms. It might be that you must look for it or get the information from the hospital but, once you start you will see there is a world of help and information out there. Places such as Macmillan will welcome you, listen to you and guide you. I have listed on the back reference pages just a few places that I know of, but I urge people not to shy away from talking about this and if you do notice anything different with changes in your body, whether it be a lump, a skin discoloration, mole, or your body not functioning as it should, then please get it checked out and seek advice.

See reference pages at the back of this book

A piece written by my Dad on behalf of my parents: -

Cancer is a disease mentioned in everyday conversations, but you do not expect it to come knocking at your door, especially your children's.

Jackie spoke to my wife and myself about a problem she had and made an appointment to see her doctor. From this an appointment was made to have scans and blood tests at the hospital and a further appointment to see the doctor with the results. On that day, my wife and myself went with Jackie and was taken into the consultation room to see the doctor, with a Macmillan support nurse in attendance. The doctor said to Jackie, "I am going to tell you what you didn't want to hear, you've got cancer".

I looked at Jackie expecting a flood of tears, but I was wrong, she sat there with a note pad and pen and started asking questions: What stage is the cancer at? What is the success rate? The questions rolled off her tongue and as the doctor answered the questions, Jackie wrote them down on the pad. The doctor asked Jackie if she had taken in what she had just told her and she said, "yes I've got cancer and I will beat it". I think we were all amazed at her calmness and positivity. When we got home, we had a hug and a tear but then got on with the job of facing up to it.

All through Jackie's treatment she has been so positive, bubbly, and always smiling. Her attitude has helped my wife and I to deal with this problem a lot better. The support that Jackie has had from family, friends, her bosses at work, her work mates and others who know her has been great, and of course you cannot get through this without the fantastic medical staff such as doctors, Macmillan support nurses and the advanced medication which you get now. I cannot thank all these people enough.

There is one thing that you have got to have and that is determination, which Jackie has had right through her ordeal. She has faced up to this problem with amazing courage and positivity and my wife and I sincerely believe this has got her through what surely has been a tough time for Jackie.

Tony's Story

I was aware that my sister, Jackie, had an interest in photography a few years ago, and she was keen on taking photos at events for people. Also, she had run the Great South Run in support of cancer research as she had some family members that sadly passed away from cancer and leukaemia. She felt she wanted to raise money to help towards eradicating this awful disease. She was fortunate to have Macmillan allow her to take photos at the Great South Run on their behalf. It was a great experience for her taking pictures of all those amazing people running in support of fantastic causes like Macmillan, and some having challenges of their own, too. But my story really begins when on a July evening in 2016 I had just arrived at a charity race night with friends. I had just got to the event when I felt my phone beep in my pocket. As I glanced down, I saw it was from Jackie, and the message looked quite long. I did not really pay much attention to people turning up to the event, as reading my sister's text message she started talking about tests that she had been having at Southampton hospital for a few weeks up until then. Reading on she wrote about the devastating news that the tests proved positive for an aggressive form of ovarian cancer. I was in a state of shock and confusion not knowing what to say or do.

Putting on a brave face I had to get through the evening without getting too upset in front of friends. I agreed to phone Jackie the day after when we had more time to discuss her situation and make more sense of it; and so, began the chemo and medicine sessions at the hospital. With the help and support from the Macmillan department she spent that year going through the trauma that thousands of people go through every day. For all the times she had been there to help her friends and family out, it was now our turn to help my sister get through the biggest challenge of hers and our lives. The plan was to have a few chemotherapy sessions followed by a major operation, then some more chemo to hopefully finish off the cancer. The doctors and Macmillan staff were amazing throughout the whole ordeal.

And following the months of tests and chemotherapy medication we were finally given the news that Jackie's cancer was gone. The relief was unimaginable, and we could not thank the staff, family, and friends enough for their support. This is something that you really do not think will happen to you or your immediate family.

,I and two cousins, decided that on October 2017 we would take part in the Great South Run to raise money for Macmillan in support of what this wonderful charity do for many people across the country, and of course Jackie would be there to take photographs for the charity.

One thing that really stuck in my mind on that day after following an injury in training, I had not prepared properly for the race. So, I had to walk some of the route in pain. But on the final straight, two miles from the finish, I began limping along. And despite all the encouragement from the crowd, I was cold and in pain and found it hard to keep running. But a hand from a fellow runner touched my back, and a voice said, "remember who you're doing this for". Because written on the back of my vest was the most important person who I was running this race for......"my sister". I was an emotional mess at that point. But I mentally picked myself up, ignored my insignificant pain, and jogged to the finish line in a time much quicker than I had planned. I could not thank that fellow runner enough for that encouragement, even though I did not know him, we both had our reasons for taking part, and he recognised mine.

A truly magical day.

* * *

Chapter Twenty

Superheroes

Throughout this book I have talked of my past and of people whose stories have touched me in some way.

We have lost precious family, friends, and neighbours to cancer and some are still with us on an ongoing journey. With an illness like cancer, once you get it, whether it be once, twice, three times or more, it never leaves you. The fear is there but you learn to live with it.

There are people in the public eye who inspire me for different reasons, as well as new people I have met on my journey. Some in "the cancer club", and others who use their status or wealth to fundraise or donate to help many others. I admire people like this for what they do and how they cope and bounce back in life. I could probably write a book alone just on them and although I didn't want this book to be a name-dropper, it felt necessary to share a few stories to give the reader an insight to what kind of people have helped me directly and indirectly throughout and given me the "Umph" I needed to deal with cancer. There will be those who will inspire you too along your path. When reading about people in the media who go through cancer or spend their time and energy helping charities, it highlights to us, that none of us face this alone and it can happen to anyone, no matter who you are. Whether you are famous or not, rich, poor, good, or bad, we all still have our own problems in life and for me, it is these stories that have played a role in making me the determined person I am in all this craziness and having the willpower to get up in the mornings and live.

My family, friends, colleagues, and hospital teams who were all there for me day in and day out - they are by far my biggest superheroes. They do not need capes or magic powers to be superheroes, they just need to keep being the awesome caring and uplifting people they always have been.

Having cancer has opened many new doors and relationships for me. It is like being in a new little club, not that I chose to be in this 'club', but it has made me realise there is always someone else going through just as much as me, if not worse.

These people are all surviving and fighting as best they can, and we each could not do this without the help of the oncology team, the Macmillan nurses, the surgeons, the consultants, in fact, every single person who works at the Southampton General Hospital and the Princess Anne Unit. So, from the bottom of my heart I thank these people for keeping me alive to make more memories with my loved ones, because if it wasn't for them, I would not be sitting here typing this to you now.

I loved the TV programme, Stand Up To Cancer – The Full Monty. This was televised over two nights and showed a lead up documentary followed by a strip tease stage show performed by the celebrities to raise cancer awareness.

The first night was performed by the men and the second by the women. This was such a poignant and emotional programme to watch, as it touched on these celebrities' experiences with cancer. Throughout the programme they talked openly about cancer and how it has affected them, they spent time learning the routine before their big night, and then they braved it to strip to a live audience and bare all right at the end. It was all done tastefully and certainly got the attention of the public viewers. This show was made with the aim of encouraging people to talk more about cancer and to go and get tested. Coleen Nolan from the seventies pop group the Nolan Sisters, was on board with this.

Before I found my love for Duran Duran's music, I grew up with the music of the Nolan Sisters. After school I would get my friends together to sing their songs and make up dance routines. We would have the tape cassette playing in the garage and pretended we were making a music video. I later got a standing ovation at school in a talent show singing one of the Nolan's hits 'Attention to Me'.

When I first saw Coleen Nolan on the daytime TV show, Loose Women, it brought back many childhood memories for me. Coleen was involved in the Stand Up to Cancer programme as she had lost her sister Bernadette to cancer. Being such a fan, and at the peak of their singing career, my mum decided she wanted to do something special for me.

Coleen's sister, Anne, and her husband, Brian, went through a traumatic time with the birth of their baby girl, Amy, and Anne came close to death's door. I remember even at the young age of eleven how Anne's story affected me in a big way.

Mum said nothing to me and took the time to write to Anne's husband, Brian at his football club in Torquay, Devon, in the hope he might receive it. Mum took a chance and was not expecting to hear back.

Anne made a call to my mum quite soon after receiving her letter and between them arranged for us to go meet her and baby, Amy, in Devon whilst there holidaying. I also saw her again with the rest of the band backstage at a concert they put on at the Southampton Gaumont (now the Mayflower Theatre).

Although the Nolan Sisters were a childhood band of mine, I still felt very emotional years on hearing the sad news of their sister, Bernadette Nolan's passing after she battled with cancer. I never thought it would bring out so much emotion in me, but I guess something that was a big part of my early life still hurts at such news.

The football player, John Hartson, was another brave person to get involved with the Stand Up to Cancer show. John had testicular cancer and his story reduced me to tears because of what he went through. John found a couple of lumps in his testicles yet left it four years until he got checked by a doctor. The only reason John went to see his GP was because he was suffering with continuous headaches. Because John had ignored the very first signs and had left this for so long, the cancer had been festering and spreading throughout John's body over this time.

The scary thing for me about this story is that the cancer started in John's testicles and if he had gone to his GP straight away, this could have been resolved quickly. However, he did not, and the tumours grew, and the cancer travelled right up through his body as far as his brain. This all happened within that four-year period, and as I keep repeating myself, we are all different and this could have happened to someone who could have died a lot sooner. So, as you see, if this man had dealt with this sooner, he probably would not have endured the many treatments and operations throughout his entire body and to his head. Although the cast involved in Stand Up To Cancer all had their own stories to tell, I found John's story very moving and pleased he and the rest of the cast were able to share their experiences on television. Just his story alone is one particularly good reason why you cannot leave things like this to fester in your mind or your body. You cannot leave it and think it might be nothing and go away. If you do leave things like this, then you could end up in a similar situation to John or worse.

The ladies on the daytime TV chat show, Loose Women, talked of the Stand Up to Cancer televised show. The thing that shocked me most was that quite a few of the hosts on Loose Women have each lived their individual nightmares with cancer. When something so big and ugly affects a person's life in the entertainment business, it sheds so much awareness on the subject. Those women have certainly been through the mill and are brave in the fact they are happy to talk through their stories and share their emotions and experiences on the show. Televising a programme about cancer shows us all how important it is to know your body, get checked, and how very normal it is now to talk about cancer and share knowledge. It does scare people but, is not something to be ashamed of or to keep silent about.

I grew up loving the eighties movies and music, and a lot of my heroes stem from that era. Through the media we all read or hear of famous icons who have experienced cancer or give their time and money to charities. Although the entertainment industry can seem like this wonderful lavish lifestyle (and most of the time it probably is), I think it must be difficult for anyone in this profession when dealing with life's blows in the constant limelight. People like this who face cancer with the added pressures and still get on with life, give people like me the willpower to get up and face the world head on and keep trying.

All these stories just show how much cancer is around us. From my family to the many women just on one TV show. From people in the music and film industry, to the people who I have met thanks to a chance meeting in my life, like the boho-chick and the lady with whom I had an emotional moment with at my Look Good Feel Better afternoon. Then I met Gill during my chemotherapy treatments, now a friend who I still meet up with from time to time. It is very unfortunate we lose many to this terrible disease, but there are so many success stories, and it is these I hold on to.

In the road my parents live in, there are only seventeen houses, yet I can count a handful of those people that I know of whom have endured their own cancer experiences. Some sadly are not with us, yet there are those who are still on their personal journeys living life because their treatment is working for them. My parents have neighbours either side of them who both developed cancers. One neighbour had relatives visit with a young lad called Max who was diagnosed with cancer.

Max's story is a remarkable one. His life has been a struggle for him from such an incredibly young age. Max had a tumour in his chest wall weighing 2.2lbs. Due to time constraints, he underwent a day-long operation to have one of his lungs removed, plus chemotherapy on top of this, not knowing if he had a future.

There came a stage during all of this when he told his dad he did not want to be here anymore. To hear of this young child speaking these words to his daddy broke my heart, yet you see him now running around playing football in the street like any other healthy child. Max's situation is ongoing because the tumour cannot be removed from his lower neck/top of shoulder. Although the tumour he has now is benign, this unfortunately has, and will continue to be, a part of his life with checks to the hospital. I think of Max's courage and what he is doing to lead as normal a life as possible, and I pray that a cure will be found very soon and, in his lifetime, to help him and others who go through this.

Jamie, who lived the other side was also diagnosed at a younger age with a rare type of cancer called Ewing's Sarcoma. He had a tumour on the base of his spine, and this kind of cancer affects the bones, or tissue around the bones. Jamie is still here today as living proof that this disease, in most cases, can be beaten or managed with medication and continued research. Jamie endured treatment to rid him of this, yet he is another person who has stood up to cancer. He is now a family man and when I visit my parents from time to time, I can hear his kids laughing and playing next door. This makes me smile to know that he came out the other side and life still goes on for him.

The statistics are currently that one in three people get told they have cancer, and although this looks likely to be heading towards two in three people, there are also many new maintenance drugs being certified for the market and money being raised by people to help ongoing research to find that cure. The science has come a long way as we have various drugs now that we never had around ten or so years ago. I guess I am one of the lucky ones in the fact that although there is still no cure for cancer, there are drugs I can keep using to help maintain it. There is hope.

War in The Blood was another TV programme aired which I found fascinating. A consultant named Ben Carpenter spoke of the science around leukaemia cell trials. Certain cells called Car "T" Cells which are part of the body's immune system, normally attack non-cancerous intruders such as viruses within the body. However, the T Cells do have the ability to target a specific protein, and therefore can be used to attack cancer and prevent DNA replication/gene mutation. These blood cells can be taken out and reprogrammed, to then be put back into the human body, and once injected back in, the cells travel around the body looking to find the cells affected by the cancer. The reprogrammed cells attach themselves to the cancerous cells and kill them off. Science is just remarkable and so are the people who continue to research to find a cure.

* * *

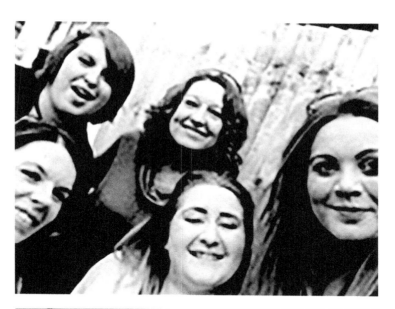

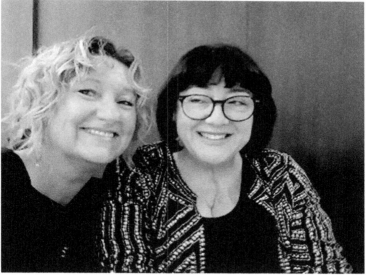

Top: My friends I met through work who kept me grounded through all the chaos happening around me
Bottom: Jo, once my manager and now a good friend. She is a treasure.

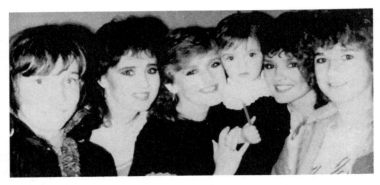

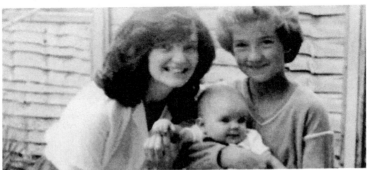

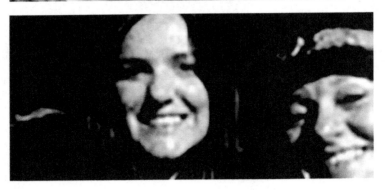

Top: *Meeting the Nolan's backstage at the Southampton Gaumont.*
Middle: *At Anne Nolan's home meeting her new-born Amy and feeling completely star struck.*
Bottom: *Tess, She has been to hell and back, yet she is one who inspires me to live life and make each day count.*

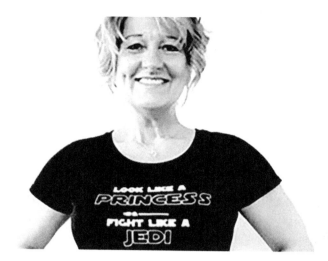

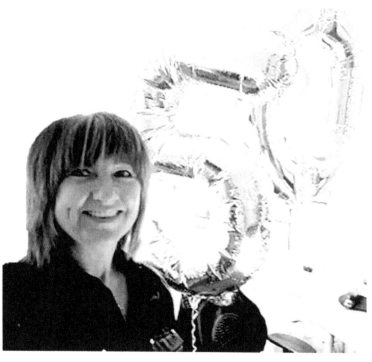

Destination 50! … and still going strong.

Epilogue

As I conclude the end of this book, I am thankful I have made it this far and for each day I wake up on this earth. We each come into this world on our own, and we each leave on our own. It is how we choose to live and deal with life that matters.

Dealing with cancer has been the toughest road I have ever taken. Yes, I live with it, but I take daily drugs to control it. I dealt with cancer in a way I never thought I would, and I had the strength I never knew was within me. I believe in the ongoing research, and I stay hopeful that one day there will be a cure.

When I started this book, I used to think of my ordeal as a fight; however, my feelings have since changed. Cancer is not a battle to win, but something I had to endure physically and mentally to live. Cancer has been the biggest life changing experience for me, and I have managed to reach my fifties feeling stronger and more empowered than I have ever felt before. I feel overcoming such challenges has made my life more meaningful and purposeful. I am using my experiences to channel all my thoughts, fears, and knowledge into this book, and I hope it will be a powerful tool to give support to others to help them get through their own personal challenges.

I strive to carry on as one of life's little miracles and my purpose for writing this book is to be the heartbeat, the sunshine, the inspiration, and the hope for others to hold on to. I appreciate not everyone is able to cope, but if you are given a chance to do something about it and you can use treatments to try and get rid of the cancer, then it has got to be worth a shot right?

I took that chance and I conquered once. Never did I think I would have to do it twice, but I did, and I will again if I must.

A beautiful person called Laura, once told me her dad always said that difficult roads lead to beautiful destinations. My difficult road has brought me this far to my destination, my fiftieth birthday. This book and my photography have been my outlet and the things that free my mind of all the cancer clutter building up.

I look in the mirror at the scars to my body from all this. Scars from my major operation and chemo treatments. I may look like damaged goods, but my heart is still in the right place, and this has given me a different perspective moving forwards. Journaling my story and turning it into this book has been a great outlet for my emotions. Cancer does scare the living daylights out of me, but still I reflect, I am thankful, and I continue to look forwards.

Then there are my personal scars by choice, my tattoos. These represent my strength, my courage, my zest for life and that which has not broken me. They represent the love, and support of my family, friends who were there protecting and encouraging me, and my medical guardian angels who have been by my side every step of my journey, and I could not have done this without them.

These tattoos remind me of how far I have come, where I am now, and how far I can continue to go in my life.

They show who I am - a Warrior Princess who stands undefeated.

* * *

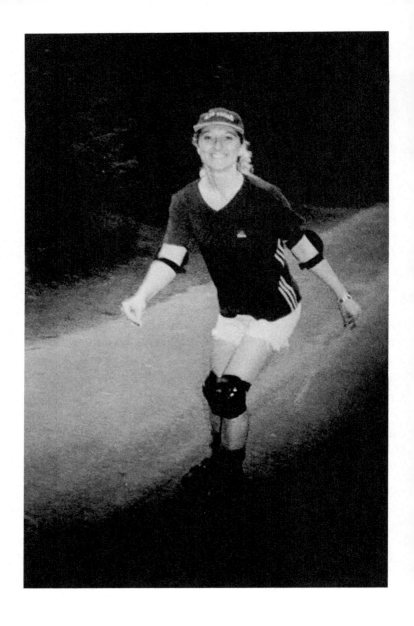

Reference pages – these are suggestions based on my experience to help those affected by cancer:

Reference 1 – my suggestions on what to take to chemotherapy treatment.

- Bottled Water, although provided by the hospital, is a must! Always take a bottle with you and keep constantly hydrated as this will help with the times the nausea might wash in and out.
- Snacks: I was advised there could be a loss of appetite as well as the nausea and to just eat whatever I felt like eating to keep my strength up and combat this. I personally believe sugar feeds cancer, but during treatment, I ensured I had my healthy snacks and took some sweet foods, too, such as fruit, ginger biscuits, hard boiled sweets, and the odd naughty item such as a bag of M&M's, chocolate bar or flapjack.
- Boiled eggs with spinach pot
- Raw vegetables/carrot batons with hummus dip or a flavoured mayonnaise
- String cheese for protein
- Crisps
- Vegetable smoothie
- Cottage cheese and rye bread
- Lucozade/fizzy drink to help aid sick feelings of the drugs being infused into me
- Ginger also helps aid sickness. Ginger biscuits or slices of ginger in green tea
- Herbal/decaff teabags and coffee as these dehydrate you less
- Sandwich
- Cooked chicken in a tub
- Cheese and crackers

Home comforts - write a list prior to your appointment and then pack what you need the evening before or on the morning of treatment:

- Kindle or reading/crossword books
- iPad/laptop with downloaded music, films, DVD's, Netflix/headphones
- Comfy clothing = "layers" = sleeveless tee shirt/hoody or cardigan/sweatpants/casual loose clothing
- Large sanitary pads in case of discharge/leaking of saline during treatment
- Pillow – should be provided by the hospital
- Dressing gown/shrug/blanket, cosy socks/slippers, sleep eye mask,
- Hand & body cream, lip balm – your skin may become dry with treatment,
- Hot water bottle = good for back if you get uncomfortable from being sat too long in chair
- Journal/note pad and pen
- Face spritz/wipes/Anti-bac gel
- Sick bag = supplied by the hospital
- Personal comforts: photo of loved ones/religious item or piece of jewellery
- Extra set of under pants, soft sports bra, or non-wired bra for comfort
- Any meds you take and pain killers = I always carry Paracetamol and Ibuprofen, but the hospital do provide these

Reference 2 – finding local support groups and charities in your area for help and advice.

For me, using these websites as a starting point to get advice and ask questions I had about my situation, benefitted me a great deal, and from there prompted more questions which I then posed to my medical team.

I believe the charity route is a better way forwards to getting the information you need rather than googling what cancer you have and become overwhelmed or scared by the information you read from other experiences. Although I write this book purely from my own personal experience, I want to keep this honest and positive to anyone experiencing cancer. The same with anything in life, you can read a lot of bad press out there as well as the good, but you must consider your own circumstances and try not to believe that what has happened to some people will happen to you.

Below are websites of charities, some of which I used during treatment, and still do now when I feel the need to talk, or if I am having a wobble about my illness. You can find many other charities out there willing to help, and some who specialise in certain areas for cancer such as breast or liver, and charities who support youth or teenage cancer.

- Macmillan: https://www.macmillan.org.uk/
- Macmillan Centre: if you have a cancer centre like this based at your local hospital then make the effort to check them out. Also contact Macmillan Citizens Advice. Macmillan are incredibly supportive and there to talk to about many things including financial advice, furniture, aids to help you, parking costs for hospital, use of their therapies on site at the hospital. They can also make you aware of other places to contact. Macmillan is a good cushion which support you and your loved ones.
- Jane Scarth: https://www.janescarthhouse.co.uk
- Cancer Research: https://www.cancerresearchuk.org
- Ovacome: https://www.ovacome.org.uk
- Change for Life: https://www.nhs.uk/change4life = for

health and fitness ideas
- Penny Brohn: https://www.pennybrohn.org.uk
- Turn 2 Us: https://www.turn2us.org.uk
- Marie Curie: https://www.mariecurie.org.uk/
- Cancer Support UK: cancersupportuk.org
- Wessex Cancer Trust: wessexcancer.org.uk
- Tenovus Cancer Care: https://www.tenovuscancercare. org.uk

If you have cancer and you are reading this do not think that you are alone. When you are first diagnosed, your head will be all over the place. You may not know where or how to start. If you feel you have no one to turn to or you are afraid to tell a loved one, then contact one of the charities listed in this book or google to find a cancer organization in your area. There will always be someone who can help and a friendly face you can go talk to. The majority of the people who work at these charities will understand as many of them have experienced cancer firsthand.

There are many support groups and places to have some nice relaxing therapies to help alleviate the stress. I believe in taking full advantage of any help that is out there for you, so do take the time to look around and try a couple out. That is what they are there for and they made a huge difference to me and my confidence. The people at these places have also played a part in why I am still standing here today making the most of life. USE THEM.

Sometimes a friend or family member can take your news worse than you, and although they support you, they can do it in a negative way without realising it. I have heard stories from people where their loved ones are regularly tearful about their situation or focus too much on the "what if" scenarios. DO lean on others if you need to and when they offer help, but DON'T lean on those who are constantly looking on the dark side of the situation you are in. This will drain you emotionally and could bring you down. This is not healthy in helping you in your situation or recovery. Yes, your loved ones may crumble when they first hear of your bad news and they will have their moment of shock, tears, and disbelief, as mine did. However, I chose to be positive and see it through, and I am lucky my loved ones chose to do the same with me. We kept hopeful and worked through this together.

Reference 3 - check list for hospital operation.

- Op/hospital Paperwork
- Head scarf/beanie hat
- Comfy big pants, sports bra for comfort if needed
- Large sanitary pads, medical anti-bacterial wash, wash bag, urine sample bottle
- Night wear, slippers, bed socks, dressing gown, towel, and flannel
- Shrug/wrap/thick warm blanket (as hospital gets cold at night), extra pillow
- Pens, ear plugs, reading book & glasses, mirror,
- Handbag with phone and money
- Laptop/iPad/crossword book/kindle, blanket
- Flip flops for shower/ surgical stockings are provided by the hospital
- Tissues, soft toothbrush, and toothpaste
- You will have a bedside cabinet to put your personal things in, and I feel it is better to take more as you can ask the person who brought you in to take back anything you find you don't need.

Do not give up! - Focus on the NOW

- Keep a journal of your journey
- Keep a memory box of cards and things
- Don't feel alone. Talk to your loved ones, your GP, your

hospital consultant, and the cancer charities and offload. Go on blogs to converse with other people going through a similar situation – just remember if they have the same cancer as you, that their journey still differs to yours. I cannot stress this enough.

- Make plans, try something new, and have goals and interests to focus on. Maybe a new social group, college course or try a new hobby.
- Pin inspirational quotes to your fridge
- Look to live a healthier lifestyle and treat yourself for sticking to it
- Take time out for yourself – meditation, spa/therapies/beauty treatment, music, a movie, walking, hobby, something social
- Fill your life with positive things and positive people and try to take a positive from a negative
- Listen to your body! Don't beat yourself up for having down days or even downtime to do nothing. YOU AND YOUR HEALTH ARE KEY IN ALL THIS.

Thank you for reading my story

Printed in Great Britain
by Amazon